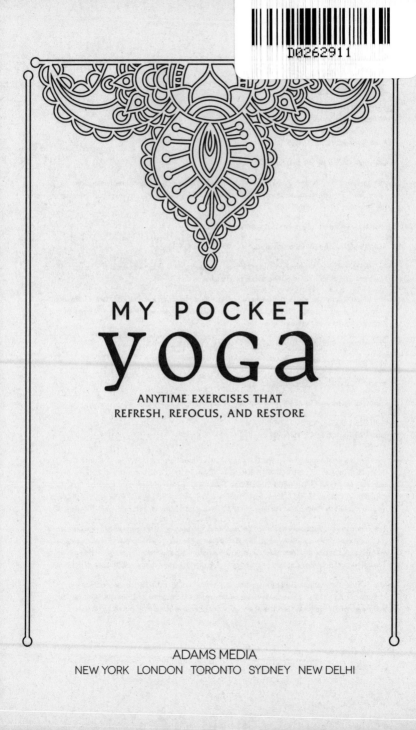

MY POCKET
yoga

ANYTIME EXERCISES THAT
REFRESH, REFOCUS, AND RESTORE

ADAMS MEDIA
NEW YORK   LONDON   TORONTO   SYDNEY   NEW DELHI

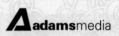

Adams Media
An Imprint of Simon & Schuster, Inc.
57 Littlefield Street
Avon, Massachusetts 02322

First Adams Media trade paperback edition JAN 2017

ADAMS MEDIA and colophon are trademarks of Simon and Schuster.

For information about special discounts for bulk purchases, please contact Simon & Schuster Special Sales at 1-866-506-1949 or business@simonandschuster.com.

The Simon & Schuster Speakers Bureau can bring authors to your live event. For more information or to book an event contact the Simon & Schuster Speakers Bureau at 1-866-248-3049 or visit our website at www.simonspeakers.com.

Printed and bound bt CPI Group (UK) Ltd, Croydon, CRO 4YY

10 9 8 7 6 5 4 3 2 1

Interior illustrations by Eric Andrews

Library of Congress Cataloging-in-Publication Data has been applied for.

ISBN 978-1-5072-0513-6
ISBN 978-1-4405-9945-3 (ebook)

Contains material adapted from *The Everything® Yoga Book* by Cynthia Worby, copyright © 2002 by Simon & Schuster, Inc., ISBN: 978-1-58062-594-4; *My Pocket Guru*, copyright © 2016 by Simon & Schuster, Inc., ISBN: 978-1-4405-9246-1; *The Everything® Essential Buddhism Book* by Arnie Kozak, copyright © 2015 by Simon & Schuster, Inc., ISBN: 978-1-4405-8982-9; and *The Everything® Guide to Chakra Healing* by Heidi E. Spear, copyright © 2011 by Simon & Schuster, Inc., ISBN: 978-1-4405-2584-1.

CONTENTS

PART 3: SEQUENCES / 123

INTRODUCTION

Looking for an easy, portable collection of your favorite yoga poses? Look no further. Whether you're new to the study of yoga or have been practicing for years, *My Pocket Yoga* will help you enjoy the mindfulness and stress-relief of yoga throughout the day. The poses, mantra, breathing techniques, and sequences you'll find in this guide will help you feel more balanced, centered, and refreshed in minutes.

You've no doubt heard about friends, colleagues, and celebrities who swear by yoga. What is all the fuss about? Yoga can help you look and feel great, open and strengthen your body, quiet and focus your mind, relieve tension, increase your self-knowledge and awareness, improve your quality of life, and change how you see the world. It has a profound and lasting effect on how you treat yourself and others. Time spent doing yoga is an opportunity to reconnect intimately with yourself on many levels and to give yourself your complete attention. When was the last time you did that?

By practicing yoga you can rejuvenate, care for, and nurture yourself at the deepest levels, resulting in greater reservoirs of compassion and tolerance for other people and a positive impact on your relationships. Most importantly, you will develop a better relationship with yourself. You will experience longer periods of calm and clarity. All those minor daily annoyances, emotional ups and downs, and responsibilities will be brought into a broader perspective, which allows them to come and go without becoming overly attached to you. You will begin to understand what is most life-affirming, beneficial, lasting, and important to you.

This book will help you become centered, calm, rejuvenated, and better able to face life's challenges, big and small. Let's get started.

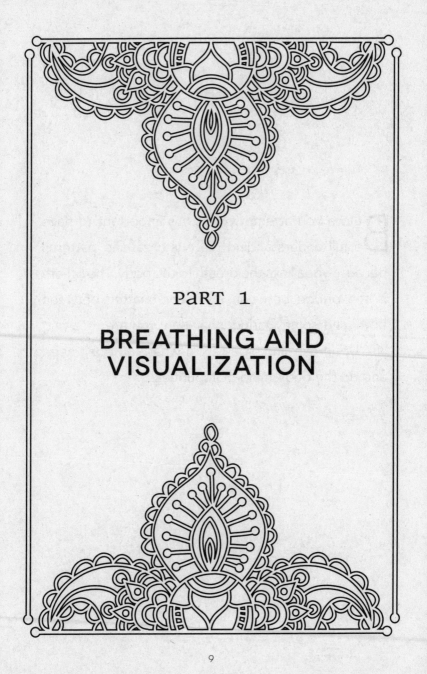

PART 1

BREATHING AND VISUALIZATION

Before you attempt poses, it's important to have a full understanding of your breathing patterns because yoga links the breath to the body. The breath is the bridge between mind and matter, between body and spirit. During inhalation, you are receiving life. Upon exhaling, you return what you don't need and rid the body-mind of impurities.

YOGIC BREATHING

When you begin practicing yoga, your respiration may be shallow, with small, fairly rapid breaths. The average person breathes sixteen to eighteen breaths per minute. As you continue your yoga practice, your rate of breath will become slower, and each inhalation and exhalation will become longer and fuller. Deeper breaths allow the energy to reach every cell.

The yoga postures open the body to receive the breath, resulting in increased elasticity of the lungs and intercostal muscles (located between the ribs). Forward bends stretch the back of the body and fill the back of the lungs; backbends open the front of the body and the front of the lungs; and lateral bends lengthen the sides of the body and the space between the lungs (the intercostal muscles). Inversions bring greater oxygen and blood flow to the brain.

In yoga, the body is considered to be a container for the life force. The nervous system is the electrical circuitry, which conducts the energy of the body. The spinal column, called *sushumna*, is the central pathway. Two other main pathways are the *pingala*, to the right of the sushumna, and the *ida*, on the left side. Balance between the ida and pingala increases the energy flow to the sushumna. The ida channel cools the body and corresponds to the parasympathetic nervous system, while the pingala heats up the body and is the sympathetic nervous system. These main channels correspond to the central nervous system and are called *nadis*. There are thousands of smaller nadis comprising the peripheral nervous system. When the energy in the body increases significantly, it is said that the *kundalini* (serpent power) energy rises up the spine (the sushumna), opening the various energy centers in the body and causing spiritual evolution within the individual.

Yogic breathing is almost always done through the nostrils. The nose is a complex and extremely efficient filtering system of foreign particles. As the breath enters the nostrils, it is moistened and warmed to body temperature. Breathing through the nose allows for deeper, fuller, and more controllable breathing.

Mouth breathing is for those times of athletic competition, such as sprint running, when the body is in oxygen deprivation because of the excessive demands being placed upon it. Then mouth breathing becomes the last resort.

BREATHING EXERCISES

Breathing is an important part of yoga. Observe your breath during the day. Check in with your breath every hour at a specified time. Slow down and tune into the quality and length of the inhalation, the exhalation, and the pauses in between. Notice if the breath is smooth or ragged, shallow or deep. Take several breaths through your nostrils and then through your mouth, observing the differences. Was the length of the inhalation and exhalation the same? Does your mouth feel dry as a result of breathing through the mouth? Which style feels more comfortable? Try the following breathing exercises as a part of your yoga practice.

Complete Breath

Lie down with bent knees, and begin breathing through your nostrils and observing your breath. Become aware of the natural length of your inhalation and exhalation, and the pauses in between. Remain relaxed without changing or forcing the breath. Let the breath flow smoothly and evenly. Relax your facial muscles and jaw.

Now place your hands on your lower abdomen, allowing them to rest there lightly. As you breathe in, feel your hands fill with your breath as your belly gently expands. On exhalation, notice how your belly contracts, moving away from your hands and receding into your body. Spend ten to twelve breaths observing the movement of the breath in your belly.

Next, lightly place your palms on your lower front floating ribs. Let your wrists relax down to your body. Again, let the breath come into your hands upon inhalation and feel your ribs contracting on exhalation. Do this for another ten to twelve breaths.

Lastly, place your hands on the collarbone and observe the breath filling the area under your hands on the inhalation. Notice how your top chest recedes with the exhalation. Practice this for ten to twelve breaths. Then allow your arms to come back to your sides, palms facing up.

Continue to watch your breath, feeling the three-part breathing pattern. You may find that the breath comes in more easily to one area than it does to another. With practice, you will be able to breathe more fully and deeply, filling your entire body with the breath.

Raising the Arms with the Breath

Stand with your feet directly under your hips. Plant your feet firmly on the floor and stand tall to lengthen your legs and spine. Have your arms at your sides, palms facing forward. Begin normal, relaxed breathing through the nostrils.

As you inhale, raise your arms slowly, feeling your belly fill up, then feeling your ribs expand and the top of your chest broaden with the breath. Let your expanding belly, chest, and ribs help you reach your arms up. At the top of the inhalation, the arms will be over your head, palms out.

When exhalation naturally starts, lower your palms as you watch the breath leave the top chest, and squeeze out of the lungs and the belly. Allow the lowering of your palms to help push the breath out of your body. Practice coordinating the lifting and lowering of the arms with the flow of the breath.

Do at least five breaths this way. Be aware of how you feel after this experience. Do you feel more grounded and internally connected? Are you calmer and more focused?

SPECIAL TYPES OF YOGIC BREATHING

The following are specific breathing exercises that will sharpen your breathing proficiency.

Pranayama

Pranayama is a powerful, ancient practice of directing energy in the body. Do this exercise if you're feeling a big draggy during the day.

1. Sit or lie down in a comfortable position, with your spine supported.
2. Close your eyes or fix your gaze softly on a still object.
3. Inhale, expanding the belly area in three dimensions. Envision the breath going deep into the belly. As you do this, imagine the lower part of your entire torso expanding in three dimensions—the side and back body as well as the front.
4. Keep inhaling, and imagine the torso expanding at the level of the rib cage.
5. Continue to inhale, expanding the chest in front and behind to the shoulder blades.
6. Finally, as you exhale, allow the chest, rib cage, then belly to soften.

Ki (Chi, Prana)

Ki is the life force or living energy that connects to all that there is and sustains our life breath. (The Chinese refer to it as *chi*, while the Hindus call it *prana*.) The following exercise helps to open up your ki passages.

1. Sit upright with your spine straight.
2. Open your mouth, relax your jaw, stick out your tongue, and pant like a dog.
3. Continue for several minutes. These in-and-out breaths will open up your belly and clear the ki passageways from the base of your spine to your throat's vocal cords.

Nadi Shodhana

One of the best-known breathing techniques for producing a calm and steady breath pattern is Nadi Shodhana, an alternate-nostril, channel-purifying, and balancing breath. To do this, you breathe in through one nostril and exhale out of the other. Then, inhale through that second side and exhale out the first.

1. Sit comfortably with the spine straight.
2. Hold your right hand in Vishnu mudra (a hand position where the thumb, ring finger, and pinky are extended and the other fingers are bent).
3. Close off the right nostril with the right thumb.
4. Softly breathe in through the left nostril.
5. At the top of that breath, close off the left nostril with the right ring finger, remove the thumb from the right nostril, and exhale through the right nostril.
6. At the bottom of that exhale, breathe back in the right nostril.
7. At the top of that inhale, close off the right nostril with the right thumb, remove the right ring finger from the left nostril, and exhale out the left nostril.
8. Repeat this pattern for a minute or two, keeping the breath soft, regular, and steady and the shoulders relaxed.

Kapalabhati Pranayama

This exercise is based on a kind of yoga breathing that is called Kapalabhati Pranayama, or "shining-face breathing." It makes your face luminous and glowing. As well, it is exhilarating and energizing.

1. Sit and exhale your breath completely.
2. Inhale and then exhale forcefully as if you are blowing out candles with your nostril breath. Do this ten to twenty times, quickly, depending on your stamina and comfort. The forceful

exhalation will draw the abdomen into your body and will cause a spontaneous inhalation.

3. It's helpful, in the beginning, to place your palms lightly on your lower belly. Then you can feel the lower abdominal area contract upon exhalation, moving away from the palms.

Three-Part Breath from Ayurveda

This exercise is drawn from the ancient Hindu system of medicine known as Ayurveda ("knowledge of life"). The Three-Part Breath is good for all three of the *doshas* (*vatta*, *pitta*, and *kapha*), which are the energies that, according to Ayurveda, compose the human body and mind in unique combinations determined at conception. When done with a focus on long, relaxed exhalations, it is especially good for calming the mind and nervous system. Avoid this exercise if you have had recent surgery or injury in your torso or head.

1. Sit tall to lengthen your spine.
2. Seal your lips and relax your forehead, jaw, and belly.
3. Begin to take steady, long breaths in and out through your nostrils.
4. Let your breath slow down so much that you can feel your belly, rib cage, then chest expand and contract with each inhalation and exhalation.
5. Take a few minutes to establish a relaxed and even breathing rhythm.
6. Next, begin to slow down and extend your exhalations, allowing them to become longer than your inhalations. To help lengthen your exhalations, gently contract your abdominal muscles as you breathe out.
7. Without straining, draw your navel back to the spine to create slow-motion exhalations.
8. Gradually build your exhalations to last twice as long as your

inhalations. Stay relaxed as you gently contract your abdominal muscles to squeeze the air out of your lungs. Breathing this way helps to release strong emotions such as anger, frustration, and impatience.

9. Continue for three to five minutes.

Ujjayii Pranayama

Breathing is key in most of these exercises. This exercise, which lowers your blood pressure and helps you concentrate your attention, is called Ujjayii Pranayama ("victorious breath").

1. Lie down on two blankets folded lengthwise with a folded blanket under your head and neck. Begin with normal breathing and relaxation for several breaths.
2. Exhale the breath completely without strain. Inhale slowly, allowing the breath to deepen. Feel your ribs expanding laterally and your chest lifting as the inhalation fills your lungs.
3. Inhale and then return to normal breathing for three complete breaths.
4. Exhale the breath completely. Resume the cycle of deep inhalation and normal exhalation, followed by three normal breaths. Repeat this pattern three times.

Dirgha Breath

When you do this breath, you welcome the breath deep into the lungs, causing the belly and ribs to expand three-dimensionally. An easy way to learn this is by lying on your back with the knees bent. Practice for one to five minutes and then evaluate the effect. You'll probably feel more grounded, calmer, awake, and clear-headed.

1. Place your hands on the belly, pressing down slightly to give a bit of resistance as you breathe in.
2. Inhale deeply, so that the hands rise as you breathe in.
3. Simply relax and exhale. Practice this a while. Then rest.
4. Place your hands over the sides of your ribs. As you breathe in, try to make your ribs expand outward, into your hands. Imagine your sides having fish gills as you breathe through them.
5. Place one hand on the upper chest and collarbones and the other on the back side of your shoulders, just below the neck. As you inhale, try to breathe so deeply that even these two areas expand.
6. Combine all three aspects of this breath. Breathing in, your belly, side ribs, and upper chest and back expand with the movement of the breath flowing into the lungs. Breathing out, you empty out.

Release and let go.

Cooling Breath (Shitalai Breathing)

Often during the day, especially midsummer, it's good to take a long, cooling breath and feel the cool and calm flow through your body. Cooling Breath (also known as Shitalai Breathing) is done by inhaling through your mouth and exhaling through your nose. This breathing practice should be done gently and without force. It is best to practice either early or late in the day, when the air is cool. Avoid this exercise if you are experiencing extreme cold or hypothermia.

1. Sit comfortably with a long spine.
2. Purse your lips, stick your tongue out, and curl it lengthwise, into the shape of a straw.
3. Inhale slowly through the straw and fill your lungs completely.
4. Relax your tongue and draw it back into your mouth, seal your lips, and exhale through your nose very slowly.

5. Repeat this cycle, inhaling though your curled tongue, closing your mouth, and exhaling through your nostrils, for three to five minutes.

If you can't curl your tongue, just keep it relaxed in your mouth and inhale through pursed lips.

Skull-Shining Breath (Kapalabhati)

This is an energizing breath that cleanses the lungs and entire respiratory tract. Skull-Shining Breath improves digestion and metabolism, strengthens the abdominal muscles, and energizes the mind.

Because this is such a powerful pranayama, there are several contraindications. Do not practice this technique if you have any of the following conditions: pregnancy; heart conditions, including hypertension; respiratory conditions; nervous system conditions; recent surgery; inflammation in the abdominal or thoracic regions; menstruation (the first few days).

Skull-Shining Breath is done by quickly and gently contracting the abdominal muscles during your exhalation and completely relaxing them during your inhalation. This results in a rhythmic pumping of the belly by alternating short, explosive exhales (expulsions) with slightly longer, and passive, inhales. The expulsions force the air out of the lungs, creating a vacuum. The release of the abdominal muscles allow for an automatic inhale to occur as the air sucks back into the lungs to fill the vacuum.

1. Sit in a comfortable position with your spine erect. Take a moment to relax your body and tune in to your breath.
2. Seal your lips, and notice your breath flowing in and out of your nostrils. Allow your breath to become steady and deep. You will be breathing through the nostrils throughout this practice.

3. Place one hand on your lower belly to help focus your attention on isolating and contracting this area.
4. Quickly contract your abdominal muscles, pushing a burst of air out of your lungs. Then release the contraction, so the belly relaxes, and allow air to passively suck back into your lungs.
5. As you repeat this, let your pace be slow and steady. Repeat fifteen times, creating a comfortable and smooth rhythm. With practice you will become more adept at contracting and releasing your belly.
6. Do one round of fifteen to thirty expulsions to start. Gradually increase to three rounds of thirty expulsions. Allow yourself to take several natural breaths in between each round to integrate the energy of the pranayama.

Lion's Breath (Simhasana)

Lion's Breath, also called Simhasana, prevents kapha accumulation in the body by stimulating the nerves, senses, and mind. It energizes the immune system, which can get sluggish for kapha types. It also relieves tension in the chest and strengthens the lungs, which are the home of kapha in the body. Avoid this breath if you have recent or chronic injury to the knees, face, neck, or tongue.

1. Sit in a comfortable position, either in a chair or kneeling on the floor with your hips on your heels. Ground your weight down into both buttock bones (also called sitz bones) and pull the crown of the head up to lengthen the spine. Take a moment to relax your body.
2. Close your mouth and notice your breath flowing in and out of your nostrils. Allow it to become steady and rhythmic.
3. Place your hands on your thighs with your fingers fanned out.
4. Inhale deeply through your nose as you draw your belly inward and press your chest forward, arching your upper back. Lift

your chin, open your eyes wide, and gaze upward at the spot between the eyebrows.

5. Open your mouth and stick out your tongue. Stretch the tip of your tongue down towards the chin, contract the epiglottis in the front of your throat (the cartilage that keeps you from inhaling food and liquid when you swallow), and slowly exhale all of the breath out while whispering a loud, strong "HAAAA" sound.

6. Repeat steps 4 and 5 four to six times. Then pause and relax. Close your eyes and let go as you feel the energy flowing through your head, eyes, throat, and belly.

Embryonic Breathing

The following exercise is based on the meditative exercises of the Taoist path and is called Embryonic Breathing. Imagine that your body is divided into three zones, called *cinnabar fields*. The lower cinnabar field extends from your navel down to your feet. The middle cinnabar field is your chest, and the upper cinnabar field is your brain.

1. Begin in standing position.
2. Take in three normal breaths, being very conscious of them.
3. With the fourth breath, take it in and pause for a moment.
4. In this brief pause, see the air vitalize the lower cinnabar field. It goes through your nose to the navel, and it continues downward to your feet. Release the breath.
5. With the fifth breath, take it in and pause for a moment.
6. In this brief pause, see the air vitalize the middle cinnabar field. It goes from your nose to your spine. Release the breath.
7. With the sixth breath, take it in and pause for a moment.
8. In this brief pause, see the air vitalize the upper cinnabar field. It goes from your nose upward to the crown of your head.
9. Relax and breathe normally.

MANTRAS

Mantras are sounds, words, or phrases that are repeatedly recited in a conscious manner. They are used as tools for focusing during meditation. The practice of repeating the mantra, silently or audibly, is called *japa* (meaning "muttering"). Mantras are meant to be repeated thousands of times so that you become deeply absorbed in the mantra's sound. Following are some mantra exercises to help you incorporate this practice into your daily routine.

Choose Your Own Mantra

1. Settle on a mantra. It can be a word or a phrase, but it should be affirming.
2. Assume a comfortable pose for meditation and begin your conscious breathing, making sure inhalation and exhalation are full and unhurried.
3. Repeat your mantra, either aloud or silently. Concentrate on both the sound of the words and their meaning.
4. Continue meditating and repeating your mantra as you feel your mind clear of debris and distractions.

So Hum Mantra

One of the simplest and most profound mantras is So Hum—"I am that I am." Meditating on this simple phrase, you penetrate your layers of protection and self-criticism. As you repeat So Hum over and over, you bring your awareness to who you are at the core: the quiet, still place. You discover simply that you exist, that you are.

1. Sit in a comfortable meditation posture. Feel your buttock bones rooted solidly. Sit up with a steady spine, without trying to straighten out the natural curves. Make sure that the top of your head is parallel to the ceiling, with the back of your neck long.
2. Take a deep inhale, and let out a long exhale. Take two more deep breaths, making the exhale longer than the inhale.
3. Close your eyes and bring your hands into prayer position at the Anahata (heart) chakra.
4. As you breathe in, imagine the syllable "So," and as you breathe out, imagine the syllable "Hum."
5. Do this several times. As you do this, make sure your jaw is relaxed. Begin to feel your entire body relaxing into this mantra.

Chakra Mantras

If you enjoy chanting one sound at a time, try chanting the sound associated with each chakra. Again, there are slight variations, so play with it a little bit until you feel the resonance in the right place:

* O as in OM for the root
* OO as in POOL for the sacral
* AH as in DHARMA for the solar plexus
* A as in SPACE for the heart
* E as in FREE for the throat
* MM as in WISDOM for the third eye
* NNG as in WING for the crown

The key words—om, pool, dharma, space, free, wisdom, and wing—are there to explain how the sounds are pronounced. These words also can be used as mnemonics, to help you remember which sound goes with each chakra. Om is for the root, and to remember it you can recall that om is the universal sound, the first vibration of physical creation. The root chakra connects you to the earth. For the second chakra, the sacral, a pool is filled with water, the element of this chakra. The third chakra is the solar plexus; its mnemonic, dharma, is connected to your will and how you create your life with that power and will.

The word *space* is the heart's element. The word *free* relates to the throat chakra; when this chakra is in balance you feel free to speak your truth. The word *wisdom* is what you can cultivate through the third eye. And metaphorically, experiencing bliss at the crown is as if you had wings. Pronounce the vowels when visualizing each chakra to bring the appropriate vibration to that energy center.

Buddhist Mantras

Mantras are often used as meditation devices by Buddhists. A mantra is basically a sound vibration. A constant repetition of a mantra (whether silent or aloud) can help to clear the mind of debris. Distractions fall away as the mind focuses on the repetitive sound. You can use a specific mantra for a specific spiritual purpose, or you can use the mantra in a general way for focusing the attention and clearing the mind.

Different vehicles of Buddhism tend towards using different mantras:

BUDDHIST TRADITION	MANTRA	TRANSLATION
Pure Land	Namo Amito	Glory to Amitabha
Tibetan	Om mani padme hum	Hail to the Jewel in the Lotus
Nichiren	Namu myoho renge kyo	Glory to the Lotus Sutra

Consider repeating one of these alongside a breathing exercise.

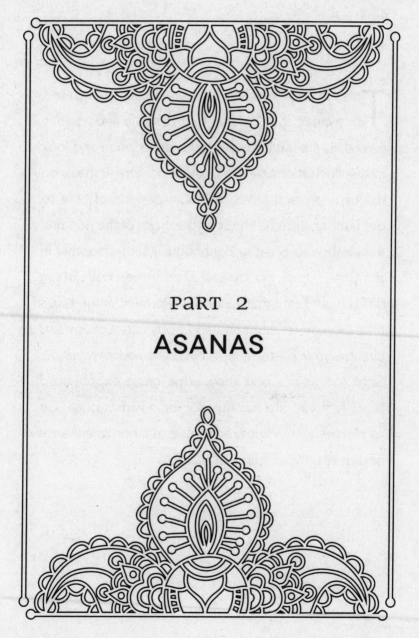

PART 2

ASANAS

This part contains nearly fifty popular yoga poses, or asanas, that you can turn to again and again in your daily life. Read through the description and look at the illustrations before doing a posture. Initially, do the pose several times for short periods of time to get familiar with the shape and actions of the posture. Remember to breathe continuously and smoothly in the pose. Don't get discouraged if the poses seem difficult at first; that's normal. Remember: It takes time to explore your mind and body connections and change your patterns of movement and perception. Seek the advice and knowledge of an experienced teacher if you are having problems with a pose. Go to classes with a knowledgeable teacher to enhance and deepen your home practice.

DIFFERENT TYPES OF ASANAS

The asanas are geometric, each with its own form and shape. In any pose, there must be a clear action, sense of direction, and center of gravity. In order to maintain the center of gravity, the muscles must be properly aligned. Stability of the pelvic and shoulder girdles is essential to the balance and symmetry of the spine.

In standing poses, the feet root down, allowing the legs and the spine to lengthen and extend away from the feet. The buttock bones are the foundation in seated poses from which the spine lifts and elongates. In inverted postures, the head, hands, or forearms provide the foundation and stability from which the torso and legs lengthen.

Remember that the goal is not the pose itself. It is the meditative process from beginning to end, which includes reflection on the effects of the asana. The asanas create different effects:

* Standing poses enhance vitality
* Seated poses are calming
* Twists are cleansing
* Supine poses are restful
* Prone poses are energizing
* Inverted poses increase mental strength
* Balancing poses create lightness
* Backbends are exhilarating

Mountain Pose (Tadasana)

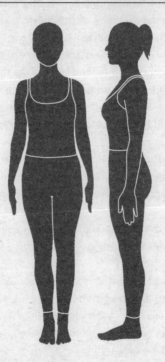

Benefits of Mountain Pose

* Teaches you how to stand correctly with proper alignment.
* Develops agility.
* Corrects minor misalignments of legs.
* Strengthens ankles.
* Relieves backache.

The Mountain Pose is the basic standing pose. Like a mountain, you want a broad, stable base from which to extend to the sky. Mountain Pose teaches you how to stand properly.

Start by placing your feet together, joining the big toes and inner ankles, if possible. Otherwise, stand so the ankles, knees, and hips are lined up, one over the other. When viewed from one side, the ear, shoulder, hip, knee, and ankle should form a straight vertical line, with your arms by your sides.

Create your yoga feet by spreading the toes and balls of the feet, pressing into the big and little toe mounds and the center of the heel. Bring the weight a little more into the heels. Lift your arches as you ground the feet. Enhance this action by lengthening your leg muscles all the way up to your hips. Lift the top of the kneecaps up by contracting the quadriceps muscle. Place your hands on your hips and extend the sides of the body from your hips to your armpits.

Bring your arms back to your sides without losing the lift of the spine and lengthen up through the crown of your head. Try to balance your head over the pelvis. Make sure the shoulders are relaxed and are not riding up to the ears. Press your shoulder blades into your back. Lift the top of your chest and broaden the collarbones. Breathe fully, balancing ease with effort. Open the body to receive the breath, remaining aware of how it feels to be in alignment.

Triangle Pose (Utthita Trikonasana)

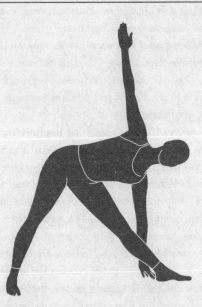

Benefits of Triangle Pose

* Strengthens and balances the muscles of the legs, hips, and spine.
* Lengthens back and abdominal muscles, providing space for the internal organs and length for the spine.
* Relieves back pain.
* Teaches sense of direction and lateral extension.
* Gives the intercostal muscles between the ribs a powerful stretch, allowing for greater lung capacity and fuller, deeper breathing.
* Expands the chest.

Begin by standing in Mountain Pose. Walk your feet four to four and a half feet apart and actively stretch your arms, from the heart to the fingertips. Feel the opening of the chest and the upper ribs as a result of the active stretch of the arms. Turn your right foot in 15 degrees and revolve your left leg out. The left foot should be at a 110- to 120-degree angle to the right foot, with the left and right heels in line with each other. The left leg is the front leg and the right leg is the back leg. Plant and spread your active yoga feet and lift the inner and outer arches up. Inhale, lengthening up through the legs and stretching them fully. Maintain the lifting of the kneecaps by contracting the quadriceps. Exhale. Elongate the sides of the body as you inhale and expand your lungs and lift the ribs. Exhale and extend laterally over your left leg, bending from the hip. Remember, it is not about how far you go down to the side; it's about being strong, extended, and balanced while moving directly to the side over the left leg. This helps keep the pose in your legs so the spine can maintain its length and freedom.

Place the right fingertips lightly on the left shin or the floor. Keep extending through both arms and equally through both sides of the body. Have the head in line with the spine and lengthen from the crown of the head to the tailbone. Look straight ahead. Try to keep the back of the body in one plane. Frequently, the upper body is leaning forward of the lower body.

Find the balance between ease and effort. Is your breath ragged or held, indicating over-effort, or is it smooth and even, indicating ease?

Maintain the pose for several breaths. See if you can continue elongating the body and opening the chest with every inhalation. Breathe normally. Inhale and come up out of the pose by grounding the feet and stretching up and back. Release the arms to your sides, bring the feet to parallel, and repeat on the other side.

Extended Hand on the Foot Pose
(Utthita Hasta Padangusthasana I)

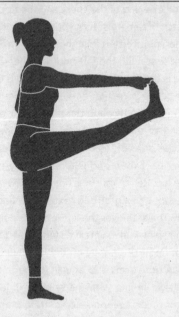

Benefits of Extended Hand on the Foot Pose

* Strengthens and tones the legs.
* Stretches the hamstrings.
* Develops balance and poise.

Stand in Mountain Pose. Transfer the weight onto the left leg and foot. Lift the right leg up and hold it outward, securing toes with your right hand. You can also place a belt around the balls of the right foot and hold the straps with each hand, or rest your leg on a chair seat or back, if that is more comfortable. Observe that the outer left hip and ankle are in line. Stretch both legs fully as you lengthen into both active yoga feet. Press down into the right heel as you lengthen up through the back of the leg and the spine to the crown of the head.

Try to keep both legs straight by the equal and opposite reactions of pressing into the feet, lifting the arches and fully stretching up through the legs, lifting the kneecaps, contracting the quadriceps muscles, and hugging the thigh muscles to the bone. Contract the quadriceps faster than you lengthen the back of the knee. Do not lock the knees, because this will cause hyperextension. Stretch the whole body up, lifting the ribs and elongating both sides of the body. Try to keep the buttocks level with each other, so one hip is not higher than the other. Stay in the pose for a few breaths. Breathe softly and fully, receiving the breath and balancing ease and effort. On the exhalation, bring the arms and leg down. Then repeat on the other side.

Extended Side Angle Pose
(Utthita Parsvakonasana)

Benefits of Extended Side Angle Pose

* Strengthens the muscles of the legs and the back.
* Opens the shoulders, hips, and groin.
* Tones the oblique abdominal muscles.
* Tones ankles and knees.
* Reduces body fat around the waist and hips.
* Expands the chest.
* Reduces sciatic and arthritic pain.
* Improves digestion.

In this posture, there is a long diagonal stretch on the upper side of the body, all the way from the foot to the fingertips. Start in Mountain Pose and jump or walk the legs wide apart to a comfortable distance (even wider than in the Triangle Pose). Extend the arms out to the sides. Turn the left foot in 15 degrees, and revolve the right leg out. Heel is in line with heel. Ground the feet, spread the toes, and lift the arches. Keeping the feet active, firm the muscles to the bone throughout the posture to keep the energy flowing, to support the knees, and to maintain a stable base of the legs and feet.

Inhale through the nostrils, infusing the body with the breath as if you were smelling a pleasing fragrance, and lengthen up through the legs and the sides of the body. This will lift and expand the chest. Exhale fully as you bend the right leg (at the hip, knee, and ankle), with the knee in line with the heel. The leg will form a 90-degree angle. Bend the torso, from the hips, directly to the side over the right leg and bring the right hand behind the right foot, fingertips touching the ground. Turn the left arm up from the shoulder. Inhale and extend the left arm up and over the head. This external rotation of the left arm flattens the shoulder blade on the back and opens the chest.

As you firm the outer edge of the left foot down, lengthen up the left side of the body into the fingertips. Look straight ahead, with the chest facing forward, keep the head in line with the spine, and observe the marvelous diagonal stretch you have created on the left side of the body. Stretch into the crown of the head and into the tailbone. Continue breathing naturally and smoothly.

Elongate the right side from the hip to the armpit. Keep the shoulder blades on the back. Feel the opening and stretching of the pelvis. Stay in the pose for a few breaths. Keep reaching. Come up out of the pose pressing into the right foot, lengthening the right leg, and reaching out the left arm. Turn the feet back to parallel, and then repeat on the other side.

Revolved Side Angle Pose
(Parivritta Parsvakonasana)

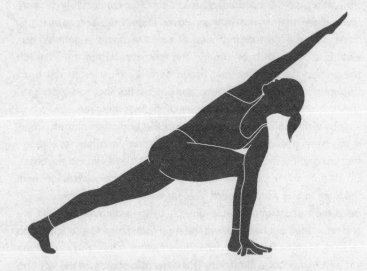

Benefits of Revolved Side Angle Pose
* Aids in digestion and elimination as it contracts and wrings out the abdominal organs.
* Gives the back muscles a powerful diagonal stretch.
* Loosens the hips and shoulders.
* Trims the waist and abdomen.
* Relieves sciatic pain.
* Reduces arthritic discomfort.

Begin by standing in Mountain Pose. Walk or jump the feet wide apart. Extend the arms from the heart to the fingertips. Turn the left foot way in, 45 to 60 degrees. Turn the right leg out so the foot is at 90 degrees. Inhale the breath, and on the exhalation turn to face the front (right) leg. Inhale and extend up from the grounding of the feet into the fingertips. Exhale completely and bend the right leg. Bend forward from the hips and turn your whole body to face your right leg.

Press the left fingertips down on the floor by the outside of the right foot and extend the arm into the shoulder socket. Place the right palm on the small of the back. Lengthen the spine as you inhale and further revolve the body around the spine as you exhale. Keep the head in line with the spine. When ready, extend the arm up and over the head. Otherwise, leave the palm on the small of the back.

Do not force or strain in the twist. Relax the effort somewhat and then see if you can twist a little more. Breathe. Mindfully come out of the twist as you exhale. Plant the feet firmly, and fully firm and stretch the legs as you bring the body upright. Bring the feet to parallel, center the body, and release the arms down. Repeat on the other side.

Half-Moon Pose (Ardha Chandrasana)

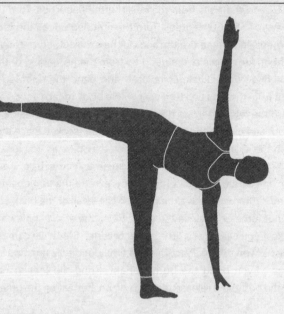

Benefits of Half-Moon Pose
* Helps balance asymmetry of the sides of the body.
* Strengthens weak muscles and stretches tight muscles.
* Elongates the spine.
* Strengthens the hips, legs, knees, and foot arches.
* Stretches the hamstrings.

To begin, stand in Mountain Pose. Walk your feet wide apart. Raise and extend the arms out to the sides. Turn the left foot in 15 degrees and revolve the right leg out. Inhale and lift the ribs and on the exhalation come into the Triangle Pose. Pause for a moment and enjoy the pose. Look forward throughout the pose, instead of turning the head to look down. Place your left hand on your hip and keep it there.

As you reach out with your right hand, bend the right leg to a right angle and place the fingertips of the right hand firmly on the floor, several inches in front of the right toes. Simultaneously walk the back leg towards the front. If your fingers do not reach the floor, use a block to bring the floor to you.

Press into the right foot, stretch the leg fully, and draw the standing leg muscles up to the hip socket. At the same time, lift the left leg up parallel to the floor. Pull up the standing leg kneecap. Extend through the left heel and balls of the foot to maintain energy and firmness in the leg. Repeat on the other side of the body.

Intense Side Stretch Pose (Parsvottanasana)

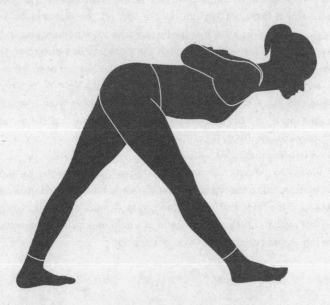

Benefits of Intense Side Stretch Pose

* Improves balance and coordination.
* Lengthens the hamstrings and the back side of the body.
* Opens the hips.
* Tones the abdomen.
* Cools the brain and calms the nerves.
* Relieves arthritis of the neck, shoulders, elbows, and wrists.
* Improves digestion.
* Tones the liver and spleen.
* Reduces menstrual pain when practiced before and after (not during) menstruation.

This is an asymmetrical forward bend that stretches each side of the body separately. The chest receives an intense stretch. Stand in Mountain Pose. Jump or walk the feet wide apart. Place the hands on the hips. Turn the left foot in 45 to 60 degrees, and turn the right leg out. Inhale the breath, grounding the feet, lifting the arches, and bringing the inhalation and extension all the way up the legs and the body. Lifting the ribs away from the hips, maintain the lift of the quadriceps and the hugging action of the leg muscles throughout the pose.

Exhale and turn to face your right leg. Place the hands in reverse prayer position behind the middle back. Revolve the left leg in its socket, turning the front thigh to face forward (without strain or force). Inhale and extend the spine, looking up. Exhale and, bending from the hips, swing the body over the right leg. Gaze at your toes. Lengthen from the crown of the head to the tailbone. Maintain a long, concave spine.

See if you can balance the forward action of the torso extending over the front leg by pulling your hips back, and drawing the top of the thighs and the hamstrings behind you. Then you will be moving in two directions, creating space throughout the spine. If you only move forward, you will lose your balance and fall forward. If you can bend more deeply in the hips and maintain the length created in the spine, bring your head towards your shin.

Try to keep the feet grounded and draw the thighbones into the hip socket. Simultaneously level the hips by pulling the outer right hip back and releasing the left hip forward to help you turn the hips even more. Stay in the pose for a few breaths and then come back up by pressing strongly into the feet with strong legs, and a long spine. Repeat on the other side. Place the back heel on the wall if you need additional support.

Standing Forward Bend (Uttanasana)

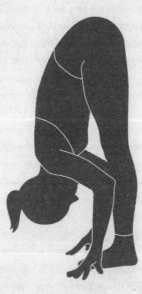

Benefits of Standing Forward Bend

* Reduces stomach discomfort.
* Strengthens the back muscles and the hamstrings intensely.
* Relieves mental and physical exhaustion.
* Slows down the heartbeat.
* Tones the liver, spleen, and kidneys.
* Decreases abdominal and back pains during menstruation.

The Standing Forward Bend is an intense stretch of the hamstring muscles and a lengthening and strengthening of the back muscles and the spine. Stand in Mountain Pose. Inhale the breath, root down onto the feet, stretch up through the legs, and elongate the spine as you contract the kneecaps and the quadriceps muscles to help the hamstrings lengthen. Firm the thigh muscles as you lift up through the crown of the head.

Roll the upper inner thighs and groin muscles back, keeping the lower back broad. Draw the shoulder blades into the back to lift and open the chest. Maintain active yoga feet and a strong lift of the inner groin muscles and legs. Actively lift and stretch your side ribs and spine up and over as you exhale and bend forward, folding at the hips.

Let the arms come down towards the floor. Place the fingertips on the floor in front of the feet. The legs draw up so the spine can release down. Breathe and allow the effects of gravity to release the back muscles, spine, and head down. Contract the kneecaps and the quadriceps muscles to help the hamstrings lengthen. Broaden the backs of the calves and the backs of the thighs.

When you are ready to come up, press the feet down and keep the legs really active, so that the strength of the thigh muscles support the stretch of the hamstring. This will prevent the feeling of locking the knees (hyperextension of the knees, pressing the knees back). Look forward, lengthening the crown of the head and the tailbone away from each other. Inhale and come up with a concave back.

Standing Half Forward Bend
(Ardha Uttanasana)

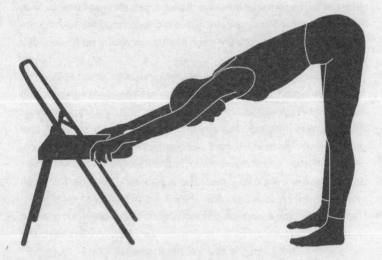

Benefits of Standing Half Forward Bend

* Fully stretches the back side of the body.
* Lengthens the spine and teaches alignment.

Stand in front of a chair. Bend over to place the hands on the sides of the chair seat and press the hands into the seat. As the hands root into the chair seat, stretch the arms back into the shoulder socket. Remember, for every action there is an equal and opposite reaction. The elbows are firm and straight. Continue lengthening from the shoulders to the buttock bones, making the sides of the waist long. Keep the shoulder blades in contact with the back body and back ribs. This stabilizes the shoulder joint and helps to open the chest. Even in a forward bend the chest remains open and the spine remains long. This action will help keep the spine happy, whereas the legs should do the most work in the pose so the spine receives the action.

The upper body is parallel to the floor, with the head between the arms. The neck and head are in line with the spine. The crown of the head stretches forward as the tailbone lengthens back. The heels are in line with the buttocks and the feet are hip width (or wider) apart. Tight hamstrings require a wider leg stance. Maintain active yoga feet and legs.

Chair Pose/Fierce Warrior (Utkatasana)

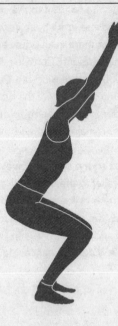

Benefits of Chair Pose/Fierce Warrior

* Strengthens the back, legs, ankles, shoulders, and arms.
* Eases shoulder stiffness and expands the chest.
* Lifts the diaphragm and gently massages the heart.
* Develops stamina and endurance, especially for skiing.

Stand in Mountain Pose and separate the feet hip width apart. Bend the hips as if to sit down. Also bend the knees and the ankles as deeply as (comfortably) possible. Ground the feet and slightly draw your weight back into your heels, so they receive most of the weight. This makes the action felt in the thighs rather than the lower back, since the legs are doing the work, and it is better for the health of the back.

Pressing down into the active yoga feet, descend the buttocks, inhale, and stretch the arms up. Lift the frontal hipbones up away from the thighs. The thighs will do most of the work in the pose—there will be sensation to confirm this. The area around the ankles will feel a good amount of stretch and action. Groin muscles and abdomen remain soft and recede into the body.

Lengthen into the fingertips, connecting this action with the lifting and stretching of the side ribs up, while drawing the upper-arm bones back into the socket. Lift the top chest to help move the shoulder blades into the back. Look straight ahead and breathe. Feel the expansion of the chest area. Monitor your breath, looking for ease and smooth regularity of the inhalation and exhalation. To come out of the pose, exhale, and release the arms down to the sides as you press the feet into the floor and lift the kneecaps and quadriceps to lengthen the legs back into Mountain Pose.

Revolved Triangle Pose
(Parivritta Trikonasana)

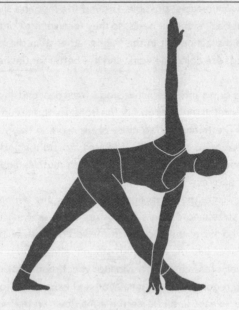

Benefits of Revolved Triangle Pose

* Develops balance and coordination.
* Provides a long, diagonal stretch of the torso muscles from shoulder to hip and wrings out the body organs.
* Expands the chest.
* Strongly works the legs.
* Strengthens the hip muscles.
* Eases back pain.
* Reduces fat around the waist and hips.
* Decreases sciatic pain.
* Reduces arthritic pain.

Stand in Mountain Pose and jump or walk the legs wide apart. Inhale, raise, and extend the arms actively out to the sides. Turn the left foot in 45 to 60 degrees and revolve the right leg out so the foot is at 90 degrees. On an exhalation, turn the body completely to face the right leg. Revolve the back (left) leg so the front of the thigh faces forward. Turn towards the right as you extend the torso, and place your left hand on the floor by the outside of the right foot. Place the right palm on the lower back. Continue revolving the torso around the axis of the spine as you extend from the crown of the head to the tailbone. Then extend the right arm up, stretching into the fingertips.

To help with balance, press strongly into your active yoga feet and draw the hips and upper thighs back behind you to balance the forward movement of your body. Draw the kneecap, quadriceps, and hamstring muscles firmly up the leg.

Inhale the breath, hug the muscles to the bone, and with strong legs come up out of the pose, taking care not to lose the grounding of the feet as you do this. Turn the feet back to parallel and the body back to center. Release the arms down to the sides. Pause and reflect, then repeat on the other side.

Warrior I (Virabhadrasana I)

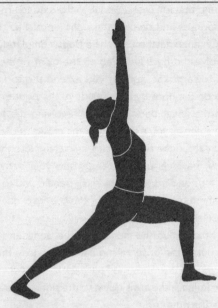

Benefits of Warrior I

* Develops balance and coordination.
* Develops strength in the legs.
* Opens the groin.
* Stretches and tones the abdomen.
* Increases stamina.
* Improves digestion.
* Relieves backache.
* Strengthens the bladder.
* Corrects a displaced uterus.
* Strengthens the back muscles.
* Relieves menstrual pain and decreases heavy periods when practiced before and after (not during) menstruation.

This is a vigorous posture that provides a tremendous stretch to the torso, the spine, and the back leg. Begin by standing in Mountain Pose. Jump or walk the legs four feet apart. Extend the arms out to the sides, palms facing up. Stretch into the fingertips and feel the opening of the chest and ribs. Inhale and lift the arms up over the head.

Connect the stretch of the side ribs with the lifting of the arms. Keep the palms facing each other, lengthen the arms, and firm the elbows. If the elbows bend, bring the arms wider apart, in the shape of a V. By straightening the elbows, you will enhance the lifting of the side ribs and the extension of the spine.

Turn the left foot in 45 to 60 degrees and revolve the right leg out. On an exhalation, turn your body to face the front (right) leg. Ground through the feet, lift the arches, and extend all the way from the feet to the legs, the side body, and the fingertips. Relax the top of the shoulders away from the ears to maintain the length of the neck and to release shoulder tension. Keep the eyes, face, and throat soft. Inhale the breath for extension, and as you exhale, bend the right leg (knee over ankle) and lengthen the left leg, pressing the top of the left thigh back. Don't worry if the left heel comes slightly off the floor. Lengthen the left leg from the hip to the heel. Bend the right leg, with the intention of creating a right angle. Continue to stretch from the side ribs into the fingertips to maintain lift and extension in the body.

Stay for a few breaths. Observe your breath. Is it even and smooth, indicating stability and ease? Is it ragged or are you holding the breath due to overexertion?

Come out of the pose by pressing the feet firmly into the floor, carefully lengthening the front leg, turning the feet to parallel, facing center, bringing the arms down, and jumping the feet back to Mountain Pose. Repeat on the other side.

Warrior II (Virabhadrasana II)

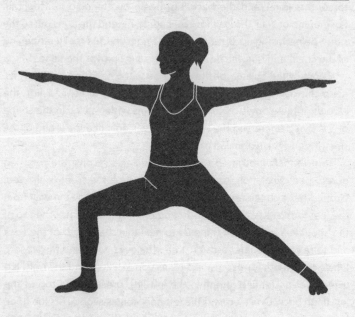

Benefits of Warrior II

* Teaches coordination of movement and breath, as well as correct alignment.
* Increases strength in the abdominal, back, buttock, and leg muscles, which contribute to the support of the spine.
* Tones the abdomen.
* Stretches and opens the legs, pelvic girdle, and buttocks.

Warrior poses create strength of body and mind. Inhale and jump or walk the feet wide apart. Lift and extend the arms out to the sides from the center of the body to the fingertips throughout the pose. Open and lift the chest as you inhale. Keep the chest expanded and lifted throughout the pose. Turn the left foot in 15 degrees and revolve the right leg out 90 degrees, heel in line with heel. Press the feet firmly down.

Inhale the breath and create extension in the body from the feet up to the fingertips. Exhale fully and bend the right leg to a 90-degree angle, with the knee over the ankle. The entire leg bends to achieve this, not just the knee. The hip, knee, and ankle bend. The right thigh descends down towards the floor. (If you cannot get into a 90-degree angle, don't worry; just do the best you can without force or strain.) As the right leg bends, the left leg remains long. The left foot actively grounds, especially on the outer edge of the foot. The left kneecap lifts up as the quadriceps muscle contracts.

There is a dynamic interplay and balance between the action of the legs. As much as the right leg bends, that's how much the left leg straightens through extension and grounding. Become aware of this duality and try to maintain a balance between the two actions.

The arms continue to extend out from the centerline of the body with the shoulder blades pressing into the back, supporting the upper body. The body remains centered between the legs. To achieve this, stretch even more into the left arm and fingertips, so the body remains upright.

The tendency is for the body to lean towards the bent leg. This causes undue strain to the right knee. Imagine that someone is holding on to your left hand and pulling you out of the pose.

Maintain the length and extension of the torso. Lift the rib cage away from the hips, and descend the hips. Feel the space created in the abdomen and the lower back. Gaze towards your right hand and remain for several breaths. To come out of the pose, look forward, press down into your right foot, lift the kneecap and quadriceps up to lengthen the right leg, and turn the feet parallel. Repeat on the other side.

Wide-Legged Forward Bend
(Prasarita Padottanasana)

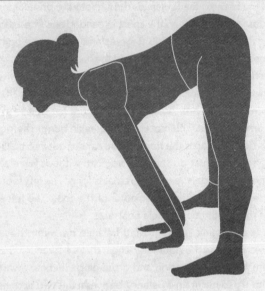

Benefits of Wide-Legged Forward Bend

* Opens the hips.
* Increases blood flow to the upper body and the head, and is good preparation for the headstand.
* Fully stretches the hamstring muscles.
* Strengthens the adductor (inner thigh) muscles.
* Improves digestion.
* Is a good substitute for those unable to do the headstand.

Stand in Mountain Pose and jump the feet wide apart. Place the hands on the hips. Make the feet parallel to each other. Spread the toes as you press the soles of the feet down and lift the inner and outer arches up. Rebound the action up the legs, lifting the kneecaps, firming the quadriceps, and hugging the leg muscles to the bone. Lengthen the sides of the body away from the hands (on the hips) all the way up to the armpits. Press the shoulder blades into the back to open and lift the chest. Breathe and expand the lungs out to the side ribs.

Inhale the breath. As you exhale, fold forward from the hips, maintaining the length of the spine you have just created. Place your fingertips on the floor (or your palms, if flexible), shoulder width apart, either in line with the toes or in front of the toes. The arms are fully stretched, with the upper arms drawn up into the shoulder sockets. Keep the length of the spine. The front, back, and sides of the body remain elongated and the back is concave.

Look straight ahead, lengthening into the crown of the head and into the tailbone. Keep breathing, and on an exhalation, fold deeper into the hip crease and let the head and spine hang down as the tailbone lifts up. Let the elbows bend back towards the legs as the palms come down to the floor.

Maintain the feet and leg action throughout the posture and keep the weight in the legs, so the spine can be free. Stay for a few breaths, breathing fully without strain. Then inhale and look forward, straightening the arms and again lengthening into the crown of the head and the tailbone. Exhale. Place the hands on the hips and stamp the feet down, activating the legs even more. Lift the shoulders up and the tailbone slightly away from the floor, and look forward. Create a long spine to come out of the posture. Release the arms down to the sides.

Bound Angle Pose (Baddha Konasana)

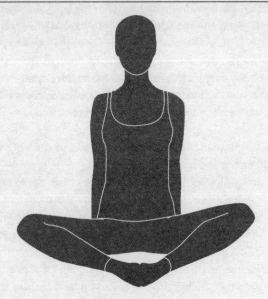

Benefits of Bound Angle Pose

* Stretches the inner thighs and groin muscles.
* Opens the pelvis and lower back.
* Reduces sciatic pain.
* Maintains healthy kidneys, prostate, ovaries, and bladder.
* Is a wonderful pose for pregnancy, helping with delivery and diminishing varicose veins.
* Eases menstrual discomfort.
* Is recommended for pranayama and meditation practices.

Sit evenly on the buttock bones with the legs outstretched and together, in front of you. Bend the knees out to the side and join the soles of the feet. Press the soles of the feet together, pressurizing the balls of the feet and the heels while you peel the toes away from each other. Observe what this feels like. What actions do you observe in the legs? Check in with your breath.

Using the hands, draw the feet in towards the pelvis, to where it is comfortable. Let the thighs release down to the floor. Open the soles of the feet, with your hands, as if they were the pages of an open book. Place the fingertips on the floor behind the hips. Press into the fingertips and stretch up through the arms. This will lift and lengthen the spine and the sides of the body. Inhale and press into the buttock bones. Elongate the spine all the way to the crown of the head. Exhale fully and lift the top chest, keeping the shoulder blades on the back. Remain for several breaths. Join the knees together and come into Four-Limbed Staff Pose. You may want to sit with the back against the wall for support.

If you suffer from knee pain, refrain from doing the pose and try the Seated Wide-Angle Pose.

Easy Pose (Sukhasana)

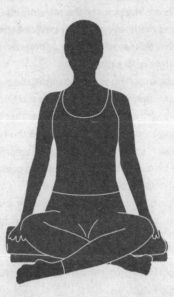

Benefit of Easy Pose

* Is well suited to meditation and breathing practices.

Sukhasana is the sitting pose we Westerners refer to as sitting crosslegged. Sit on one or several blankets with your legs crossed at the ankles. With your hands, roll the inner thighs down to the floor and then draw the buttocks flesh diagonally back behind you to broaden your base and lengthen the groins. Ground the buttock bones equally as you exhale. Inhale, and let the thighs release down to the floor. Lengthen up through the sides of the body. Place the hands by the hips, and, as in the Four-Limbed Staff Pose, lift the buttocks off the floor slightly, and then lightly place them back down, maintaining a long torso. Lift and expand the chest. Put the palms on top of the thighs, closer to the hips. Lift and open the top chest. Gaze straight ahead for several breaths. Release the pose, change the cross of the legs, and do Sukhasana again.

Head-to-Knee Pose (Janu Sirsasana)

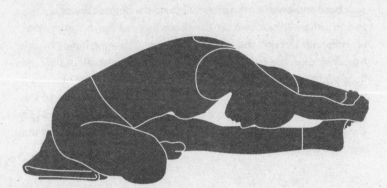

Benefits of Head-to-Knee Pose

* Improves digestion.
* Tones and stimulates the kidneys.
* Stretches the back side of the body and legs (one at a time), relieving stiffness and strengthening the leg muscles.
* Decreases stiffness in the shoulder, elbow, wrist, and finger joints.
* Results in hip opening for the bent leg hip.
* Lengthens the spine.
* Increases knee flexibility.

Begin by sitting evenly on the buttock bones with the legs outstretched and together, in front of you. Bend the right leg out to the side. Holding on to the back of the knee, draw the knee back to a comfortable position. Place the sole of the foot by the inner-left thigh. The left leg is extended, with the center of the back heel on the floor. The left foot is actively spreading, inner and outer arches are lifting, and the balls, joints of the toes, and heel are stretching forward.

Turn the body to face the left leg. Clasp the outer foot or hold on to the outer shin with the hands. Turn the navel to face the inner left leg. Press down evenly with the buttock bones, the back of the left leg, and the right thigh. Lengthen up through the sides of the body. Draw the upper-arm bones back into the sockets to open and lift the top chest.

Enhance this action as you make the back concave, which creates more length in the spine. Inhale, and on the exhalation, bend from the hips and extend the body out over the extended left leg. Lift the ribs away from the hips. If you are more flexible, the arms may bend with the elbows out to the sides, causing the chest to remain wide. Repeat on the other side.

Sideways Wide-Angle Pose
(Parsva Upavistha Konasana)

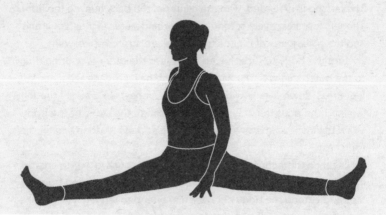

Benefits of Sideways Wide-Angle Pose

* Relieves backaches.
* Tones the abdominal organs.
* Tones the kidneys.
* Stimulates blood and lymph circulation.
* Opens the hips.

Sit in Seated Wide-Angle Pose. Place the right fingertips behind you and the left fingertips on the floor in front of the pubis. Press the fingertips down and ground the legs and the buttock bones as you inhale and lift the spine and sides of the body up. Exhale and gently revolve the body towards the right leg. Do this for several breaths, gently increasing the revolving of the spine and torso. Then carefully unwind back to center. Repeat on the other side.

Seated Wide-Angle Pose
(Upavistha Konasana)

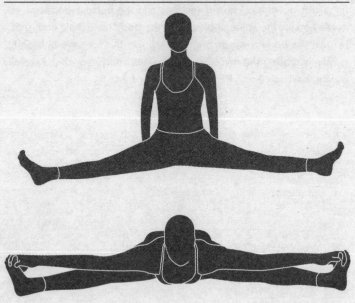

Benefits of Seated Wide-Angle Pose

* Permits full stretching of the back of the body and the legs.
* Tones the abdominal organs.
* Improves health of the reproductive organs by increasing circulation.
* Balances the menstrual cycle, stimulates the ovaries, and eases menstrual discomfort.
* Prepares the body for labor and delivery.
* Tones and stimulates the prostate gland.

Begin by sitting evenly on the buttock bones with the legs outstretched and together, in front of you. Separate the legs at a comfortable, wide distance apart. Press the fingertips down by the sides of the body to lift and elongate the torso. Lift the rib cage off the hips. Root the center of the back of the heels and the legs into the floor. The toes face the ceiling. Actively lengthen the legs in two directions, towards the feet and into the hips. Breathe and be in the pose.

To go farther in the posture, bend forward from the hips and extend the body out and forward. Maintain the elongation of the front, sides, and back of the body. Clasp the big toes or calves with your hands. The buttock bones must remain grounded on the floor. The head may reach the floor or remain extended in the air.

Seated Straight-Leg Forward Bend
(Paschimottanasana)

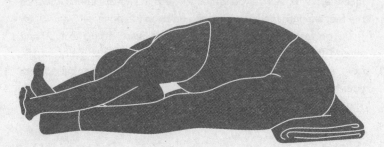

Benefits of Seated Straight-Leg Forward Bend

* Is an intense stretch for the back side of the body.
* Tones the abdominal organs.
* Improves digestion.
* Rejuvenates the spine.
* Calms and quiets the mind and the nervous system.
* Soothes the adrenal glands.
* Stimulates the ovaries, uterus, and the whole reproductive system.
* Once you are able to stay in the pose for several minutes, gives the heart a good massage and replenishes the reproductive organs.

Sit evenly on the buttock bones with the legs outstretched and together, in front of you. Press the fingertips down on either side as you lengthen up through the sides of the torso. Maintain this as you clasp the feet with both hands. Ground the buttock bones and the back of the legs. Stretch your active yoga feet out as you draw the thighbones back into the hip sockets.

Inhale, look up, and lift up through the crown of the head, creating a concave spine. Keep the sternum lifted. Exhale as you bend forward from the hips and extend the body over the legs. Lift the ribs away from the hips. Stay in the pose for several breaths. See if you can create more internal space as you inhale, and move deeper into the pose (if appropriate) with each exhale. Inhale up the front of the spine and exhale down the back. The forehead can rest on the legs or remain extended in the air. Gaze at the legs or the toes.

You can also try sitting on a folded blanket to keep the pelvis upright and neutral. Place the fingertips behind the hips as you bend forward.

Belly Twist (Jathara Parivartanasana)

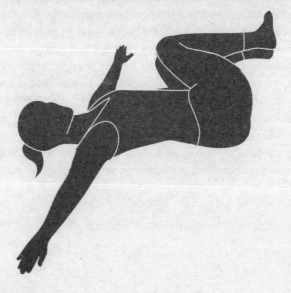

Benefits of Belly Twist

* Is a powerful, stimulating, and wringing action for the waist, abdomen, and lower back.
* Strengthens transverse and oblique abdominal muscles.
* Strengthens inner and outer thigh muscles.

For this pose, lie down and bend the knees with the feet flat on the floor. Lift the feet away from the floor and bring the knees to the chest. Extend the arms horizontally on the floor. Stack the knees and ankles and let the knees come down to the floor on the right side at a 90-degree angle. Gaze up at the ceiling. Feel the belly and the ribs spiral towards the left. Maintain the length of the spine upon inhalation, twist on the exhalation, and roll the left shoulder down towards the floor (without forcing). Stay in the pose for several breaths, deepening the twist. Then bring the knees back to center and go to the other side.

Sage Twist (Maricyasana III)

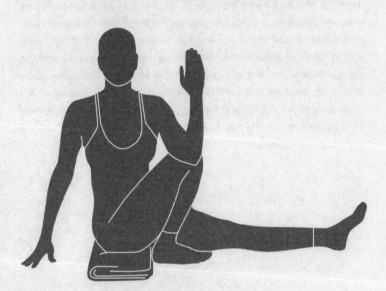

Benefits of Sage Twist
* Loosens the shoulders, lower back, and hips.
* Increases energy level.
* Improves the functioning of liver, spleen, pancreas, kidneys, and intestines.
* Eases backache.
* Nourishes discs.

Sit evenly on the buttock bones with the legs outstretched and together, in front of you. Press the fingertips of both hands onto the floor and lengthen the arms and torso. Bend the right knee and clasp both hands under the knee. Bring the knee into the chest and the heel to the right buttock bone. Firmly plant the right foot on the floor. Keep pressing the foot down throughout the posture. Extend through the left leg actively and press the back of the leg down.

Turn to the right. Wrapping the left arm around the right knee and hugging the leg into the body, place the right hand behind you. Re-create the length of the right arm and the extension of the right side of the body by pressing the fingertips down and drawing the arm up to the shoulder socket.

Inhale, extend the right arm up, and, exhaling, bring the outside of the arm against the outside of the bent knees. Press the leg against the arm and the arm against the leg to help with the revolving action of the twist. Inhale the breath and extend the spine. Exhale and spiral the torso towards the right leg. Move the right knee forward and bring the back ribs into the front ribs. Bend the right elbow and stretch the fingertips up to deepen the action and bring the shoulder blades onto the back. Do this for several breaths, gently increasing the revolving of the spine and torso. Slowly release back to center, and repeat on the other side.

Instead of bringing the left arm to the outside of the right knee, you may want to try hugging the left arm around the right knee. Inhale, lengthen the spine, and exhale, twisting while drawing the right leg into the body. You can also sit on a folded blanket to neutralize the pelvis. Place the back hand on a block. This enhances the extension of the body on that side. You can also bend the elbows to increase the twisting action and open the chest.

Twist on Chair (Bharadvajasana)

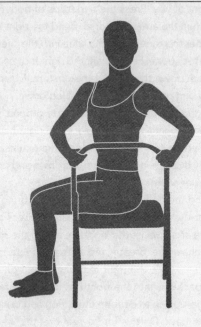

Benefits of Twist on Chair

* Relieves arthritis of the lower back.
* Improves digestion.
* Alleviates rheumatism of the knees.
* Tones the liver and kidneys.
* Increases circulation to the abdominal organs.
* Exercises the abdominal muscles.
* Increases suppleness of spinal muscles.

Sit sideways on a chair. The left side of the body is next to the back of the chair. Plant your feet flat on the floor with heels under knees. If the feet do not make it to the floor, bring the floor to you by placing a book or two under the feet.

Hold on to the top of the chair back and bend the elbows wide apart to stretch and open the rib cage, making more room for the breath to enter. Press the buttock bones down into the chair seat as you inhale and lengthen the sides of the body up. Exhale and gradually revolve the body around the spine, towards the back of the chair. With every inhalation, create lift, extension, and space in the body. After three or four breaths, carefully unwind and return to center. Repeat on the other side.

Basic Relaxation Pose (Savasana)

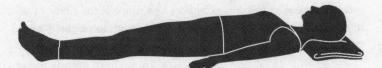

Benefits of Basic Relaxation Pose

* Soothes the nerves.
* Calms and quiets the mind.
* Diminishes migraines.
* Minimizes symptoms of chronic fatigue syndrome.
* Reduces insomnia.
* Aids in recovery from surgery or chronic illness.
* Removes fatigue.
* Integrates the effects of the asanas practiced prior to Savasana.
* Prepares you for pranayama.
* Gives you an increased awareness regarding areas of stress and tension.

Essential in yoga (as well as many other disciplines) is the relaxation of the mind and body. Yoga achieves this through the posture called Savasana. This posture also helps prepare you for breathing techniques.

1. Lie down on your back with your legs extended. Use a folded blanket under your head and neck so your forehead and chin are level with each other. Turn your palms up while rotating your upper arms outward. Have your arms rest slightly away from the sides of your body.

2. Balance the sides of the body, arms, and legs, feeling equal weight on the shoulders, buttocks, arms, and legs. Then release the effort.

3. Scan your body and become aware of how you feel. Note the quality of your breath as it becomes smooth and even.

4. Soften your eyes. Spread and soften your forehead skin.

5. Soften your ears and relax the eardrums. Relax behind your cheek muscles. Spread and soften your chin. Relax the throat muscles and soften the tongue.

6. Observe the heaviness of your body, arms, and legs as the body begins to relax and let go. Soften the diaphragm and ribs. Soften your abdomen and release your lower back to the floor.

7. Remain in this Basic Relaxation Pose anywhere from five to twenty minutes. Then deepen your next exhalation and lengthen the following inhalation. Move your fingers and toes, and stretch your arms above your head. Bend your knees and slowly roll onto your right side, and use your hands and arms to come to a seated position.

Supported Bound Angle Pose
(Supta Baddha Konasana)

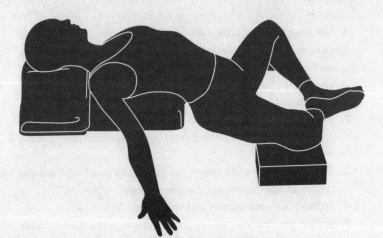

Benefits of Supported Bound Angle Pose
* Eases menstrual discomfort.
* Opens the chest, abdomen, pelvis, inner thighs, and groin.
* Deepens the breath.
* Benefits the health of the ovaries and the prostate gland.
* Regulates blood pressure.
* Relieves varicose veins and sciatica.
* Helps a prolapsed uterus.
* Tones the kidneys.

Stack one to three vertically folded blankets (one on top of the other) behind you, with the narrow end a few inches away from your buttocks. Sit evenly on the buttock bones with the legs outstretched and together, in front of you. Bend the knees out to the sides and join the soles of the feet together. Draw the heels in towards the pelvis, at a comfortable distance for the knees and hips.

Place your hands on either side of the blankets and lower your back (keeping it extended) and head onto the blankets. Let your arms come out to the sides, with the palms facing up. They will be off the blankets. Close your eyes. Relax completely. This is a wonderful restorative posture. Stay in the pose for five to ten minutes, depending upon your comfort level. Observe your breath and the expansion of the torso upon inhalation and the contraction of the body on exhalation.

To come out of the pose, bring your knees together and carefully roll off the blankets onto your right side. Press your hands down to bring yourself to a seated position.

It may be necessary to place a folded blanket under your head, so your chin is neither pressing into your chest nor sticking way up in the air. Your chin can be level with your forehead or a little lower. You want to retain the natural (concave) curve of the neck. Your legs can be propped up with additional blankets or blocks for extra support.

Reclining Hero Pose (Supta Virasana)

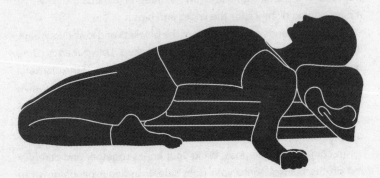

Benefits of Reclining Hero Pose
* Stretches the abdomen, waist, back, and front of thighs.
* Improves digestion.
* Opens the lungs and allows for easier breathing, providing some relief from asthma.
* Relieves menstrual discomfort.
* Reduces inflammation of the knees.
* Relieves pain in the legs and rests them.
* Enhances resistance to infection.
* Develops arches and helps correct flat feet.

Come to a kneeling position. Have two to four vertically folded blankets, one on top of the other, placed behind your buttocks. Separate the feet and sit down between them. The feet should touch each hip (as best you can). Ground the buttock bones, sitting evenly on them. Pressing down into the buttock bones, exhale, inhale, and lengthen up through the spine to the crown of the head. Stretch and spread your toes and the soles of your feet. Roll your inner thighs slightly down to the floor while spreading your buttock bones away from the tailbone, or turn the calves out. Place the palms down on either side of the blankets, and lengthen the spine out of the pelvis. Rest on the elbows, as the body lowers onto the blankets.

Remain in the pose up to five minutes, depending upon your level of comfort and ease. This is another great restorative pose. To come out of the pose, press the elbows and forearms down on either side of the blankets, and come up with the chest lifted. Carefully extend one leg at a time.

Reclining Hand-to-Big-Toe Pose 1
(Supta Padangusthasana I)

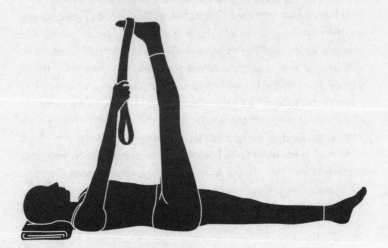

Benefits of Reclining Hand-to-Big-Toe Pose 1

* Develops the leg muscles.
* Balances the action of the leg muscles, so they work synergistically with each other.
* Lengthens the back muscles and hamstring muscles.
* Relieves sciatica.
* Increases hip flexibility and strength.
* Enhances health of the reproductive organs and provides relief from menstrual pain.

Lie down and extend the legs on the floor. Stretching into the feet, lengthen into the crown of the head. Bend the right leg and extend it up to perpendicular, with the sole of the foot facing the ceiling. Hold on to the big toe with the first two fingers or hold on to the outside of the foot.

Press the back of the left leg down. Lengthen the inner and outer heels away from the ankles, spread the toes, and lift the inner and outer arches. Feel the action drawing up the legs.

Elongate the sides of the body from the hips to the armpits. Lengthen from the right waist to the hip to equalize both sides of the body. The right side will want to shorten because of the leg being raised. Avoid this by maintaining the length on both sides of the body. Stay in the pose for several breaths and then lower the leg and repeat on the other side.

Reclining Hand-to-Big-Toe Pose 2
(Supta Padangusthasana II)

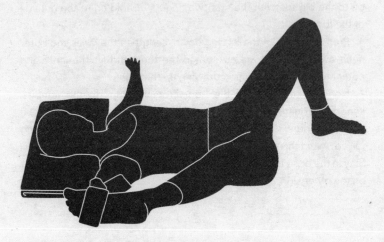

Benefits of Reclining Hand-to-Big-Toe Pose 2

* Develops the leg muscles.
* Balances the action of the leg muscles, so they work synergistically with each other.
* Lengthens the back muscles and hamstring muscles.
* Relieves sciatica.
* Increases hip flexibility and strength.
* Enhances health of the reproductive organs and provides relief from menstrual pain.

Lie down and raise the right leg to perpendicular. Place a belt around the outstretched leg and hold onto the strap with the same hand as the raised leg. Bend the bottom leg, foot flat on the floor, to make it more comfortable for the hamstrings. Place the bottom foot against a wall for enhanced stretching of the bottom leg. Fully stretch the legs throughout the pose. On an exhalation, lower the right leg down to the right side. The hips must remain level with each other, so the leg may not reach the floor. Look at the ceiling. Remain in the pose for a few breaths and then carefully raise the leg back up to perpendicular, release the grasp of the hand, and lower the leg to the floor. Repeat on the other side.

Restorative Bridge Pose
(Setu Bandhasana Sarvangasana)

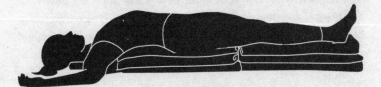

Benefits of the Restorative Bridge Pose

* Opens the chest and expands the lungs.
* Improves quality and volume of the breath.
* Stretches the front of the body.
* Lengthens the groin muscles and stretches the psoas muscles.
* Calms and quiets the brain.
* Soothes the nervous system.
* Relieves backache.
* Increases blood circulation to arteries.
* Decreases insomnia and stress headaches.
* Improves digestion.
* Rests the legs.
* Prevents varicose veins.

This is a restorative pose, which provides similar benefits to the shoulderstand. In fact, it is good neck and upper-body preparation for shoulderstand, as it stretches the neck and opens the chest, stretching the (often) tight upper-chest muscles. Setu Bandhasana Sarvangasana can be substituted for shoulderstand during menstruation.

Place two bolsters vertically, one behind the other (or use four to six blankets vertically folded) on the floor. Lie the whole body and legs on the bolsters, so the bottom edge of the shoulder blades are on the upper edge of the bolster. The tops of the shoulders roll down to the floor, doming and expanding the upper chest. The back of the head is on the floor. The arms can be diagonally by your sides, with the palms facing up, or they can be bent at the elbows, like a cactus. The elbows will be in line with the shoulders.

Loop a belt firmly around the middle of the thighs, so they will not be able to roll apart. An extra belt can also be looped around the middle of the shins for extra support.

Close the eyes and relax. Remain in the pose from five to fifteen minutes. To come out of the pose, bend the knees with feet flat on the floor, and release the belt. Carefully move yourself in the direction of your head, until your back and buttocks are on the floor and your knees are bent (to rest your back). Then roll onto the right side and, using the hands, bring yourself up to a seated position.

Upward-Facing Dog
(Urdhva Mukha Svanasana)

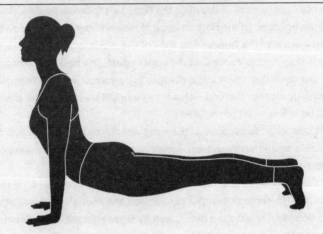

Benefits of Upward-Facing Dog
* Is a wonderful stretch in the front body and its organs.
* Improves flexibility of the spine.
* Strengthens back muscles and spine.
* Increases bone density.
* Relieves backache such as sciatica and slipped disc.
* Expands the chest and increases lung capacity.
* Improves circulation in the pelvis.

This is the counter pose to Downward-Facing Dog. It is a backbend, while Downward-Facing Dog is a forward bend. Upward-Facing Dog has similar actions to the Cobra Pose, the difference being that the legs come off the floor in Upward-Facing Dog.

Lie down on your belly. Extend the legs straight out, behind you. Place your hands flat on the ground by your waist, fingers facing forward. Stretch from the legs to the toes; hug the thigh muscle into the bone. Inhale and look forward. Extend your chest and your upper back forward and your ribs forward and up. Draw the ribs away from the belly to create space for the spine to come in, lengthen, and coil.

Press the hands and feet down to lift the legs slightly off the floor and to support the torso. Exhale the breath. Stretch into the toes as you continue coiling the spine forward and up. Bring the upper arms back and open the top chest to draw the shoulder blades into the back. Lift the kneecaps and firm the thighs. Avoid over-squeezing the shoulder blades together (creating a crease between them). The shoulder blades move into the back body. Gaze upward, if the neck is comfortable, or else look forward. Feel the stretch in the belly. Stay in the pose for several natural, smooth breaths and then come down and release.

You can also tuck the toes under instead of coming up on the front of the feet. This will stimulate muscle-hugging action in the legs. When using the arms in the pose, bend the elbows out to the sides and press the chest and upper back forward. Then lengthen the arms. Do this several times. This enhances the expansion of the chest and the drawing in of the shoulder blades against the back.

Sphinx Pose

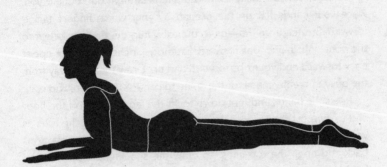

Benefits of Sphinx Pose

* Strengthens the upper-back muscles.
* Opens the chest and stretches the muscles on the front body.
* Teaches basic backbending action.

Lie on your belly with legs extended behind you. Prop yourself up on your forearms. Your forearms will be parallel to each other with the elbows close to the waist and in line with the wrists and shoulders. Press the forearms and the palms down and observe how this grounding action lifts the chest and elongates the sides of the body. Maintaining this action, pull the elbows back on the floor without actually moving them. Feel the muscles of the upper back draw in to the back and hug the shoulder blades. Enhance this by lifting the sternum forward and up. Enjoy the openness and broadness of the top chest. Stay for several breaths and then release down and rest.

Cat-Cow

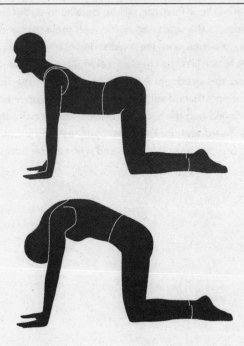

Benefits of Cat-Cow

* Increases the flexibility and suppleness of the spine and its surrounding muscles.
* Stretches and tones the muscles of the back.
* Plumps up the spinal discs and aids in fluid circulation in and out of the discs.
* Stimulates the nervous system.
* Is useful as a warm-up for other postures and as a way of stretching the back side of the body after backbending.
* Teaches coordination of the breath with movement.
* Releases tension in the back.

This pose warms up the spine beautifully, creating suppleness and stretching the back muscles. Start on all fours. Wrists are under shoulders and knees are under hips. Look forward and lengthen into the crown of the head and into the tailbone. Slightly tip the tailbone up (see Pose 1). Inhale the breath. Press the inner thighs away from each other, hugging the bone. Exhale and round the spine by curling the chin into the chest and lifting each vertebra up towards the ceiling (see Pose 2). Draw the tailbone in between the legs towards the pubis bone. The pubis bone moves towards the navel and the navel recedes and presses up to the front of the spine. Press the hands down and push the hands away from the body as you round the back. Repeat the lengthening on the inhalation and rounding on the exhalation nine more times, coordinating the movement with the breath.

Plank Pose (Phalakasana)

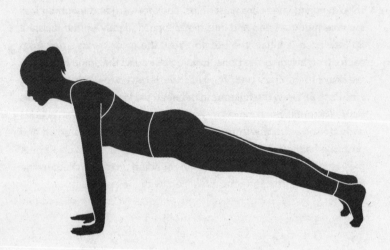

Benefits of Plank Pose

* Increases upper-body strength.
* Develops upper-back muscles.
* Is an excellent weight-bearing exercise for increasing bone density.
* Opens the chest.

Plank Pose is a weight-bearing pose, which is good preparation for other poses emphasizing upper-body strength. Lie down on your belly, bend your arms, and place the hands on the floor and under the shoulders (fingers facing forward). Extend the legs behind you and tuck the toes under. The more you walk the toes towards the legs, the more activity and muscle-hugging bone action there will be in the legs.

Press the hands down firmly and feel the upper-back muscles start contracting and drawing in to the shoulder blades and against the back. Now the actions of the hands, feet, and legs have supplied the necessary support for the Plank Pose.

As you maintain these actions, press the hands and toes down, exhale into the lower abdomen, and stretch the arms up into the shoulder sockets, lifting the torso and legs off the floor. Make sure the shoulder blades are supporting and opening the chest. Stretch the heels away from the body as the kneecaps and the front of the thighs firm and stretch towards the hips. The body, from the shoulders to the hips and feet, forms a slanted line of strength and alignment. Be in the pose for several breaths and then come down.

As in Downward-Facing Dog, you can place support under the wrist to distribute the weight into the knuckles and fingers. You can also try coming into Plank Pose from Downward-Facing Dog. Bring the shoulders over the wrists and lower the hips while stretching and firming the arms and legs, and pulling the heels away from the legs. Be careful not to let the abdomen, hips, and thighs sag, or the lower back will get compressed. If you have wrist pain, use support under the wrist. If pain persists, come out of the pose.

Salute with Eight Parts or Points
(Ashtanga Namaskara)

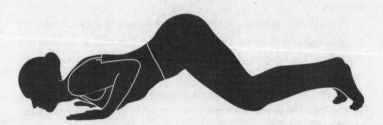

Benefits of Salute with Eight Parts or Points

* Improves back mobility.
* Increases arm strength.

Begin in Plank Pose. Exhale and extend down into the heels, rebounding down into the feet and hands to move up, stretching the sternum forward, and keeping the legs and abdominals firm. Shoulders are over the wrists and hands are on the floor. Inhale. Exhale and lower the knees, chest, and chin to the floor.

Child's Pose (Balasana)

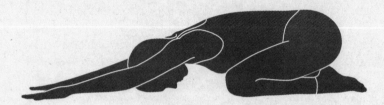

Benefits of Child's Pose
* Increases circulation in the lower back and abdomen.
* Stretches the back muscles and the spine.
* Eases lower back discomfort.
* Is a good resting pose to do between strenuous postures.

Start on all fours, with the hands under the shoulders and the knees under the hips. Inhale and on the exhalation draw your buttocks back to rest on your heels. Press the hands on the floor, extending into the fingertips, and stretching back through the sides of the body to the hips. Let the forehead rest on the floor. While in the pose, inhale and feel the expansion of the waist and lower back. Exhale and observe the contraction of the ribs and lungs as the breath leaves the body. Stay for several breaths and then come back up and release the pose.

If the head does not reach the floor, place a folded blanket under the forehead. If the buttocks do not meet the heels, place a folded blanket between the heels and buttocks for support. Walk the hands to the right for several breaths and then to the left. This stretches one side of the body at a time, and is particularly beneficial for scoliosis, where one side of the body is convex and the other is concave.

Four-Limbed Staff Pose
(Chattaranga Dandasana)

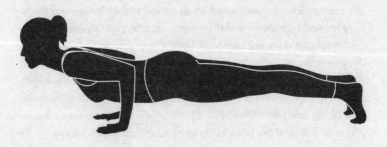

Benefits of Four-Limbed Staff Pose

* Increases upper-body strength.
* Increases bone density.
* Strengthens arms and wrists.
* Improves wrist flexibility.
* Contracts and tones abdominal organs.

Lie down on your belly with legs extended and hands under shoulders, fingers facing forward. The elbows are next to the waist, not out to the sides. Press the hands down and lift the top of the shoulders away from the floor. The goal is to have the shoulder at the same height as the elbows throughout the pose. Otherwise, the upper-arm bone will not be in the socket, and there is a possibility of injuring your neck and shoulders through misalignment. Observe the muscle action in the upper back. Feel the shoulder blades hugging the back.

Shrug the shoulders towards the ears slightly to feed the upper-arm bones into the shoulder socket. Now the arms and shoulders are supporting the upper body. Tuck the toes way under and walk them towards the body. This action helps lift the kneecaps and firms the thighs, drawing the muscle energy up the front of the leg to the hip. The thighbones insert into the hip sockets, supporting the pelvis. Now stretch the heels away from the back body, stimulating muscle action through the back side of the leg from hamstrings to heel. Feel the thighs and hips lift slightly off the floor.

Inhale the breath and as you exhale press the lower abdomen against the front of the spine, press the hands and toes down, and lift the body up, like a staff, off the floor. Lengthen the collarbones and sternum towards the head and the abdomen and lower back towards the heels. The hips and shoulders are the same height off the floor. See if you can stay up for a second and come down. Try it several times, using your breath to facilitate the movement into the pose.

This pose is not to be done by pregnant women once the belly is protruding. People with wrist problems should do the pose carefully, using support under the wrist to decrease the angle of the bend in the wrist. Distribute the body weight through the entire hand, not just the wrist. Press the fingers down as you lengthen into the fingertips. If you have shoulder problems, check your alignment. Make sure the shoulders remain in line with the elbows. Hold the pose briefly and repeat several times, unless pain is present.

Cobra Pose (Bhujangasana)

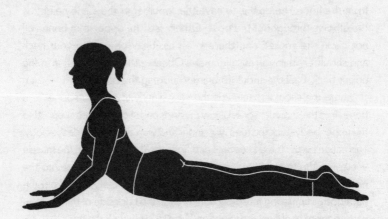

Benefits of Cobra Pose
* Stretches the front of the body and its organs.
* Strengthens the spine and back muscles and relieves backache.
* Squeezes, tones, and stimulates organs in the back body.
* When done correctly, can relieve sciatica and slipped disc (best done under the supervision of a qualified yoga professional).

Lie on your belly with your forehead on the floor, your hands under your shoulders, and your legs outstretched (together) behind you. Press the hands and the front of the feet down and lengthen the toes away from the body. Draw the elbows into the waist.

Inhale the breath and look forward. Feel the breath ease as the chest opens. Stretch the chest, the area between the shoulder blades (upper back), and the ribs forward. The ribs and the belly move away from the hips and the hips stretch away from the legs. The pubic bone remains on the floor and the lower back and tailbone lengthen away from the upper body. Space is created between the hips and the ribs, allowing the spine to lengthen into the body. The belly receives a pleasant stretch. Make sure you exhale completely.

Coil the spine into the body, like a wave that is moving in and up to arc before it spills over into the surf. Use your hands, pressing down to lengthen the arms up to support the coiling action of the spine. The arms do not have to straighten and they should not be used to create a push-up feeling (which will cause shortening of the lower back and compression). Breathe! Do not hold the breath.

Come up only as far as is comfortable for you. If there is lower-back discomfort, you have come up too far through the pushing-up action of the arms. The arms are there only to provide extra support. Stay in the pose for a few breaths and then come down. Repeat several times, going up and coming down.

Downward-Facing Dog
(Adho Mukha Svanasana)

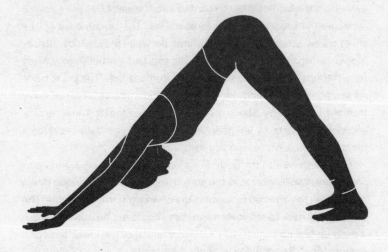

Benefits of Downward-Facing Dog

* Stretches hamstring and calf muscles.
* Lengthens the spine.
* Strengthens the upper body, arms, and wrists.
* Is great for increasing bone density as a weight-bearing exercise.
* Increases shoulder flexibility.
* Opens the chest.
* As a mild inversion, rests the heart and quiets the brain.

Downward-Facing Dog is one of the most frequently practiced yoga poses. Start on the hands and knees. Place the hands under the shoulders and the knees directly under the hips. The inner arms face each other and the elbows are straight and firm. Let the shoulder blades come onto the back. The pelvis is in a neutral position, horizontal to the floor. Tuck the toes under.

Plant the hands firmly on the floor and spread the fingers evenly apart. Press the palms, knuckles, and fingers into the floor. Especially press down the pointer-finger knuckle and balance the weight on either side of the hand.

Inhale the breath, lift the hips evenly, and press the hands and feet down. On the exhalation, straighten the legs and let the head drop between the arms. Relax the neck. Press the front of the thighs back to elongate the torso. Press the hands down, extending into the fingertips. Then stretch the arms away from the hand, all the way up to the buttock bones. Let the spine lengthen from the top of the head to the tailbone, into one long line of extension.

Lift the heels up, resisting the shoulders moving forward, and continue stretching all the way up the back of the legs to the buttock bones. Now lengthen the heels down, but keep stretching the back of the legs up. Lift the kneecaps and firm the thighs. The heels are stretching towards the floor. They might even make it to the floor, but do not force this action if it is not happening. Fully stretch the legs. Keep the arms as long as possible. Bending the elbows will make it difficult to transfer the weight of the body from the arms to the legs. Remain in the pose for several breaths, extending the spine on the inhalation. Then bend the knees and come down.

Equestrian/Lunge Pose
(Ashwa Sanchalanasana)

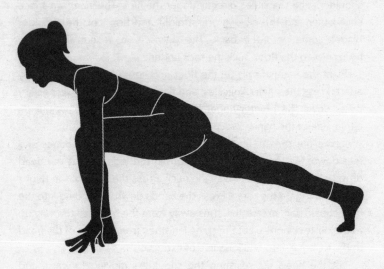

Benefits of Equestrian/Lunge Pose

* Improves range of motion and flexibility of the hips.
* Stretches and opens the groin and the psoas muscle.
* Warms up and prepares the body for backbends by opening the groin muscles.

Come onto all fours. Look forward, bend the right leg, swing it forward, and plant the right foot between the hands. Spread the toes and the balls of the feet, and lift the arches. The right shin is perpendicular to the floor, with the knee over the heel. Extend the left leg from the hip to the heel with the toes tucked under. Lift the back thigh away from the floor slightly, to ensure that the thighbone is feeding into the socket, rather than hanging out of the socket (hanging from the hip joint is detrimental to the health of the joint and its surrounding ligaments and tendons). Ground the right foot and toes of the left foot. Maintain the extension of the spine from the tailbone to the crown of the head. Press the fingertips into the floor as you stretch the arms up into the shoulder sockets to support the upper body. Be in the pose for several breaths. Then release back onto all fours. Repeat on the left side.

Pigeon Pose (Raja Kapotasana Modified)

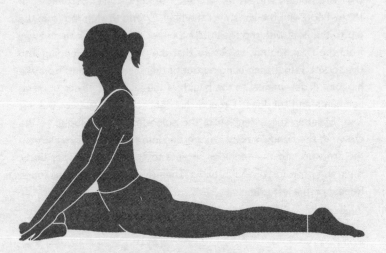

Benefits of Pigeon Pose

* Stretches the piriformis muscle located between the hip and the sacrum (a tight piriformis muscle can cause sciatic nerve pain by pressing on the nerve as it exits the sciatic notch).
* Opens and releases the external hip rotator muscles, which get tight from running, cycling, and sitting.
* Stretches the iliotibial band on the outside of the thigh.
* Readjusts the sacrum.
* Stretches the psoas muscle and the groin muscle of the back leg.

Start on all fours. Bring the right leg through as in the Equestrian/ Lunge Pose. Once the right foot is between the hands, let the right side of the leg rest on the floor. The outside of the right shin and thigh will be against the floor. Your fingertips will be on either side of the right leg. Adjust the angles of the right leg so there is some comfort in the posture. The further forward the shin is, the more intense the stretch will be on the right buttock, outer hip, and outer thigh. It is fine to bring the right heel close in towards the pubis. Tuck the toes of the back leg under to provide more muscle energy in the back leg.

Observe how you are balanced in this pose. The tendency is to sit more onto the bent leg side. Try to balance your weight between the two legs by rolling more onto the straight (back) leg side.

Prop yourself up on your arms by placing the fingertips of each hand on the floor stretching up through the arms and the spine. Let the hips sink down as if you were sitting. Stretch into the back heel. Stay for several breaths. Then come back onto all fours and repeat on the other side.

Supported Shoulderstand
(Salamba Sarvangasana)

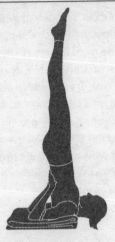

Benefits of Supported Shoulderstand

* Stimulates the thyroid and parathyroid glands.
* Increases blood flow to the heart and brain without strain.
* Opens the lungs for easier breathing.
* Is beneficial for those with palpitations, breathlessness, asthma, bronchitis, and throat discomfort.
* Soothes and quiets the nervous system.
* Relieves fatigue.
* Boosts the functioning of the immune system.
* Improves sleep quality and decreases insomnia.
* Improves digestion and elimination.
* Assists functioning of the reproductive organs.
* Regulates menstrual flow.

Stack three folded blankets on top of each other, rounded edges together facing away from the wall, a foot or so away from the wall. Lie down on the blankets, with the head and neck off the top, rounded edge of the blankets. Your shoulders should be positioned at least an inch down from the top edge of the blankets, so when you roll onto the top of the shoulders, the shoulders do not roll onto the floor. Your knees are bent with your feet on the wall at a 90-degree angle (adjust your distance to the wall so the legs can be at 90 degrees). The buttocks are on the floor. Have your arms by your sides, and roll the upper arms out so the palms are facing up.

Bend the elbows and press the upper arms down, and as you inhale lift the buttocks up. Support the lower back with the hands. The head is on the floor, shoulders are on the blankets, but the neck will be slightly off the floor. This is important for the health of the neck and for retaining its natural curve. If the neck is pressed down onto the floor, this could be injurious to the neck and could, over time and with repeated practice, cause a flattening of the natural curve of the cervical spine. Then the pose would be a neckstand rather than a shoulderstand.

Lifting the buttocks off the floor causes you to roll onto the top of the shoulders. The foundation in shoulderstand is the top of the shoulders and the upper arms. The upper arms press down, to allow the body and legs to extend up. The shoulder blades press into the back, opening the chest and drawing the upper spine into the body. The hands support the torso, but it is the back muscles and the lifting of the legs out of the pelvis that are working to hold you up in shoulderstand. Try to keep the elbows shoulder width apart and under the shoulders for alignment and support. (Tight shoulders will make it difficult to bring the elbows to shoulder width.) As you remain in the pose, see if you can move the hands down towards the shoulder blades every few breaths. Stay for several breaths, keeping the throat soft, then release the hands from the back and slowly lower to the ground.

Supported Legs Up the Wall Pose
(Viparita Karani)

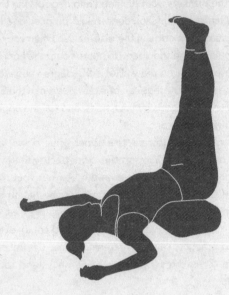

Benefits of Supported Legs Up the Wall Pose

* Drains fluid from the legs.
* Softens the belly and groin.
* Reverses the effects of gravity.
* Reverses the flow of blood and lymph.
* Rests the heart and the brain.
* Relieves tired legs.
* Revitalizes and relaxes.

Place a bolster or one to three horizontally folded blankets against a wall. Lie on your side with the left hip on the support, buttocks close to the wall, and the knees bent. Roll onto your back and swing the legs up the wall. Rest the legs on the wall, the lower back and sacrum on the support, and the rest of the torso on the floor. Have the arms outstretched horizontally with the palms facing up. The eyes may close and soften.

Breathe naturally and enjoy the relaxation and revitalization of the pose. To come out of the pose, bend the knees. With your feet on the wall, press yourself into the center of the room, with your knees bent and back resting on the floor. Then roll over onto your right side. Using your hands, press yourself up to a seated position. You can also practice Supported Legs Up the Wall Pose with your legs separated wide apart. Or you can bend your knees slightly if it is too intense a stretch for the hamstring muscles.

Tree Pose (Vrksasana)

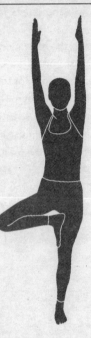

Benefits of Tree Pose

* Tones and strengthens leg muscles.
* Strengthens the ankles.
* Improves balance and coordination.
* Opens the hips.
* Lengthens the spine.
* Expands the chest for fuller breathing.

The Tree Pose develops balance and upward stretch, much like a tree, which has a strong, extensive root system, allowing it to grow tall and branch out.

Start by standing in Mountain Pose. Gaze straight ahead with a soft but focused gaze. Shift your weight to the left leg, root down, spread the balls of the feet, broaden the heels, and press firmly down with the big toe and little toe balls of the feet and the center of each heel. Turn your right foot out to the side. Then bring your right foot up to the inside of the left leg to where it is comfortable. You may use your hand to help bring the foot up the leg. Press the sole of the right foot against the inside of the left leg, leg against foot, as if they were pressing the spine up. If the foot does not easily stay on the leg, it is fine to leave it on the floor, turned out, with the right heel resting against the inner heel of the left foot. Maintain the grounding in the left foot and the extension in the left leg, taking care not to hyperextend the leg. Press the neck of the big toe down and lift the kneecap. Extend the arms out to the sides, with the palms facing up. Stretch all the way from the centerline of the body to the fingertips. On an inhalation, take the arms up over the head, stretching from the side ribs to the fingertips, palms facing each other.

Continue breathing through the nostrils, relaxing the throat and diaphragm and softening the front ribs and belly. Balance ease and effort. Stay in Tree Pose for several breaths, or as long as you feel comfortable and can maintain the pose. To come out of the pose, exhale and release the arms to the side as the right leg comes back into Mountain Pose. Repeat on the other side.

Eagle Pose (Garudasana)

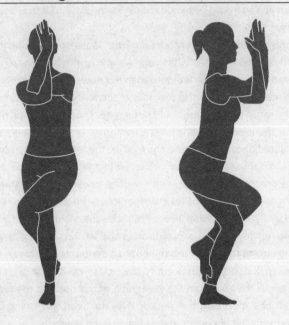

Benefits of Eagle Pose

* Improves circulation by squeezing and wringing out the arms and legs.
* Relieves shoulder stiffness.
* Strengthens the ankles.
* Helps reduce and prevent cramps in the calf muscles.

Garuda was an eagle deity in Indian mythology. To begin this pose, stand in Mountain Pose. Extend the arms out to the sides. Bring them to the center and entwine the arms, crossing the left elbow over the inside of the right elbow. Turn the palms to face each other and join them. Lift the elbows to shoulder height and move the forearms away from the face to bring the wrists over the elbows. Bend the hips, knees, and ankles as if you are sitting. Cross the left leg over the right thigh. Press the toes and balls of the left foot down on the floor. On an exhalation, lift the left foot off the ground and wrap the left shin and foot around the right calf as best you can. Gaze straight ahead. Observe your breath coming into and expanding the space between the shoulder blades. Remain in the pose for several breaths and then return to Mountain Pose. Repeat on the other side.

If your balance is precarious, keep the foot on the floor. If the hands do not join, hold on to a strap with each hand. You can also practice with your back lightly against the wall for support.

Locust Pose (Salabhasana)

Benefits of Locust Pose

* Creates a long curve of the spine.
* Strengthens the entire back side.
* Stimulates the spleen and the pancreas.

This is a prone backbend, which gradually arches the back. Lie on the belly, with the legs together and extended. Stretch into the toes. Reach the arms out in front on the floor, with the palms facing each other. Stretch into the fingertips. Inhale the breath, exhale as you firm your abdominals. Keeping the abdominals firm, inhale, lift, and extend the arms and legs. Keep breathing and lengthening into the fingers and toes. Think of lengthening your front body without shortening your back body. The head should be between the arms and at arm height. If the head is higher than the arms, the back of the neck will be shortened. After several breaths, exhale and release the pose. Rest on your belly with your head to the side. Repeat two more times.

Bridge Pose (Setu Bandhasana)

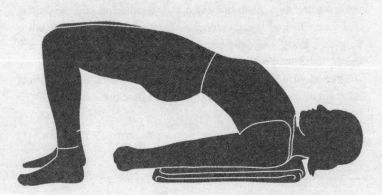

Benefits of Bridge Pose

* Is good preparation for shoulderstands and backbends.
* Increases flexibility of the spine.
* Stretches the front of the body, including the groin and thighs.
* Lengthens the back of the neck.
* Strengthens the back of the body.
* Stimulates thyroid and parathyroid glands.

Lie on your back with the knees bent and feet flat on the floor, a little wider than hip width apart. The arms are bent next to the waist, with the fingers stretching up to the ceiling. Palms face each other. Press the upper arms down for grounding to provide extension and length for the side ribs. Press the feet down as you lift the hips slightly off the floor. Do not tuck your pelvis or press the pelvis up aggressively, as this will compress and jam the lower back. Imagine that the shape of the pelvis resembles a hammock.

As you press the feet down, try to drag your heels back to your shoulders without actually moving them. This action will contract your hamstrings, lengthen your quadriceps muscles, and keep the strain out of your lower back. Support the lifting of the hips with the hamstrings and avoid overgripping of the buttocks. Breathe and stay in the pose for several breaths. Release and come down with a neutral spine. Relax and then repeat the pose.

Standing Backbend Pose (Anuvittasana)

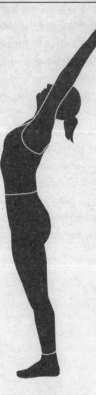

Benefit of Standing Backbend Pose

* Releases tension in neck and shoulders.

Stand in Mountain Pose with your feet hip width apart. Ground the active yoga feet and firm the thighs. Inhale, extend the spine and the arms forward, and come up with a concave back and long legs. Raise the arms over the head, look up, lift the heart, and arch the back. Exhale and return to Mountain Pose.

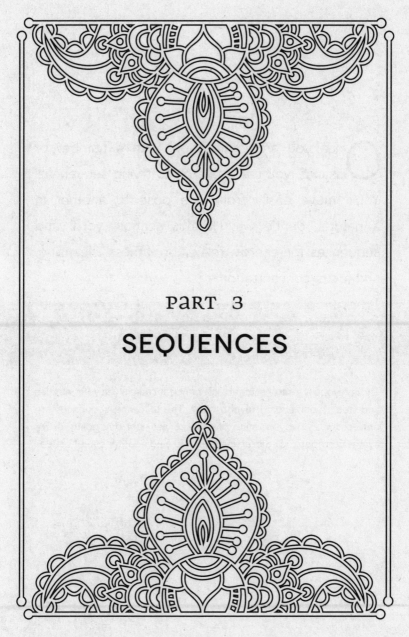

PART 3

SEQUENCES

Once you are comfortable with a number of asanas, you can move on to trying sequences. You'll move easily from one pose to another in a natural, gentle way. In this section, you'll find sequences for energy, relaxation, fitness, cleansing, and focus/concentration.

YOGA SEQUENCES FOR ENERGY

Though yoga is a serene, quiet experience, it can enliven your muscles and boost your energy level as well. The following sequences are perfect for an early-morning practice to get your day going, or for a late-afternoon pick-me-up instead of having another cup of coffee.

ENERGY SEQUENCE 1

1. **Mountain Pose:** Inhale—sweep your arms overhead, ground down through the four corners of your feet, engage your core, and make this an active pose for 5 full breaths (30 seconds).

2. **Standing Backbend Pose:** Inhale in Mountain then exhale, Standing Backbend—bend at your elbows, open your chest to the ceiling, and engage your abdominals for 3 full breaths (20 seconds).

3. **Mountain Pose:** Inhale and rise back up to Mountain for 2 breaths. Squeeze your thighs together, tuck your tailbone down, and relax your shoulders away from your ears (10 seconds).

4. **Standing Forward Bend:** Take one more breath in Mountain then exhale, Standing Forward Bend—bring your palms through heart center as you fold your torso towards your thighs and release your fingertips to your mat. Take 5 full breaths while allowing your head to hang heavy, and bend into one knee and then the next to warm up your hamstrings (30 seconds).

5. **Standing Half Forward Bend:** Inhale—place your palms on your shins or thighs, create a flat back, and breathe here for 5 full breaths. Work to parallel your torso to your mat and draw your shoulder blades together and down your back. Keep your gaze straight down (30 seconds).

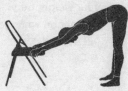

6. **Plank Pose:** Inhale in Standing Half Forward Bend then exhale, Plank Pose—plant your palms shoulder width distance apart, step your feet straight back hip width distance apart, and keep your core engaged for 5 full breaths. Create one line of energy from your heels to the top of your head (30 seconds).

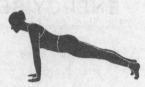

7. **Four-Limbed Staff Pose:** Inhale and shift your weight forward in Plank Pose, then exhale, Four-Limbed Staff—lower halfway down and bend your elbows up to 90 degrees for 2 breaths (10 seconds). Keep your elbows pinned into your low ribs and your gaze down.

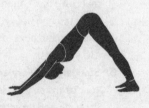

8. **Upward-Facing Dog:** Inhale—open your chest forward as you flip onto the tops of your feet. Breathe here for 5 breaths (30 seconds) and press down on the tops of your feet to engage your knees and thighs enough to lift them away from your mat.

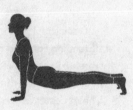

9. **Downward-Facing Dog:** Exhale—send your hips high, fold your torso towards your thighs, and send your heels towards your mat. Spread your fingers out wide and evenly distribute your weight between the four points of contact on your mat for 7 full breaths (45 seconds).

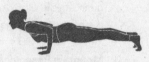

10. **Standing Forward Bend:** Inhale, look between your palms, and bend your knees; exhale, step or walk to the top of your mat, and let your torso hang from your hips. Let your arms dangle from their sockets and your head hang heavy for 5 breaths (30 seconds).

11. **Basic Relaxation Pose:** From Standing Forward Bend, bend your knees, sink your hips towards your heels, and take a seat on your mat. Slowly roll on your back one vertebra at a time for Basic Relaxation Pose—extend your legs out long and arms long down by your sides, palms facing up. Gently close your eyes and relax for 5 minutes or more.

Option: If you prefer, you can repeat the Energy Sequences at a faster pace 3 times through, linking one or two inhale/exhales per movement (5 seconds each pose). Examples:

* Inhale Mountain Pose, exhale Standing Backbend Pose, inhale Mountain Pose, exhale Standing Forward Bend.
* Inhale Standing Half Forward Bend, exhale Plank, inhale and shift your weight forward, exhale Four-Limbed Staff Pose.
* Inhale Upward-Facing Dog, exhale Downward-Facing Dog, inhale and look between your palms, exhale Standing Forward Bend.

ENERGY SEQUENCE 2

1. **Child's Pose:** Bring your big toes to touch and bring your knees to the edges of your mat. Crawl your fingertips towards the top of your mat and let your hips sink towards your heels. Let your forehead rest on your mat and spread your fingers wide. Breathe here for 10 full breaths (1 minute).

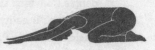

2. **Downward-Facing Dog:** Send your hips up high and fold your torso towards your thighs. Separate your hands shoulder width distance and your feet hip width distance and sink your heels towards your mat for 7 full breaths. Spread your fingers wide and press your chest towards your thighs (45 seconds).

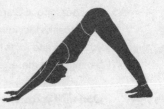

3. **Plank Pose:** Inhale in Downward-Facing Dog then exhale to Plank Pose—lower your hips in line with your shoulders and keep your core engaged for 5 full breaths. Create one line of energy from your heels to the top of your head (30 seconds).

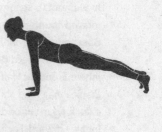

4. **Four-Limbed Staff Pose:** Inhale and shift your weight forward in Plank Pose then exhale, Four-Limbed Staff— lower halfway down and bend your elbows up to 90 degrees for 2 breaths

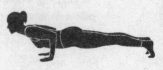

(10 seconds). Keep your elbows pinned into your low ribs and your gaze down.

5. **Upward-Facing Dog:** Inhale—open your chest forward as you flip onto the tops of your feet. Breathe here for 5 breaths (30 seconds) and press down on the tops of your feet to engage your knees and thighs enough to lift them away from your mat.

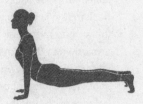

6. **Downward-Facing Dog:** Exhale, send your hips up and back, and breathe here for 5 breaths (30 seconds).

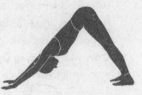

7. **Warrior II:** Inhale and raise your right leg high, then exhale and place your foot between your hands. Inhale, Warrior II—ground your back heel down, rise up, and extend your arms to the front and back of the room. Open your left hip and bend into your front knee up to 90 degrees.

8. **Extended Side Angle Pose:** Inhale in Warrior II then exhale, Extended Side Angle—reach your front arm forward and then down, and reach your back arm up to the ceiling. Continue to reach up towards your top fingertips for 5 breaths (30 seconds).

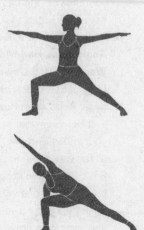

9. **Half-Moon Pose:** Inhale in Extended Side Angle then exhale into Half-Moon—launch off your back foot and bring your back foot in line with your hips. Send your left arm up to the ceiling and your right arm down to the ground. Optionally, use a block under your right hand. Stack your shoulders on top of one another and find balance for 5 breaths (30 seconds).

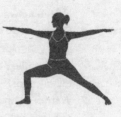

10. **Warrior II:** Inhale in Half-Moon then exhale back to Warrior II. Land your back foot down and extend your arms out in opposite directions.

11. **Downward-Facing Dog:** Inhale in Warrior II then exhale, Downward-Facing Dog—plant your palms, send your hips up and back, and breathe here for 5 breaths (30 seconds).

12. Repeat **Warrior II, Extended Side Angle Pose, Half-Moon Pose, Warrior II,** and **Downward-Facing Dog** (in that order) on the left side.

13. **Basic Relaxation Pose:** Step your feet between your hands, bend your knees, and sink your hips all the way down to your mat for Basic Relaxation Pose. Slowly roll on your back one vertebra at a time, then extend your legs out long and arms long down by your sides, palms facing up. Gently close your eyes and relax for 5 minutes or more.

ENERGY SEQUENCE 3

1. **Cat-Cow:** Place your shoulders directly under your palms, your hips over your knees. As you inhale, send your belly towards the floor and your tailbone up and gaze towards the ceiling. As you exhale, round your spine and tuck your chin towards your chest. Take 10 rounds of breath here (1 minute).

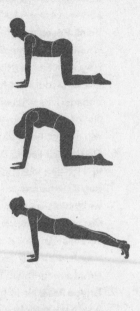

2. **Plank Pose:** Inhale in Cat-Cow then exhale, Plank Pose—curl your toes under and lift your knees in line with your shoulders. Keep your core engaged for 5 full breaths. Create one line of energy from your heels to the top of your head (30 seconds).

3. **Cobra Pose:** Place your palms directly under your elbows by your side ribs and press the tops of your feet down. Squeeze your legs together and inhale to Cobra Pose—peel your chest away from the mat and keep your gaze down to protect your neck. Breathe here for 5 full breaths with little to no weight in your palms (30 seconds).

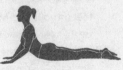

4. **Sphinx Pose:** Inhale in Cobra Pose and as you exhale release your right cheek to the mat and look left. Now bring your chin back to center and bring your elbows by your side ribs. Inhale to Sphinx Pose—press down on your forearms and palms to lift your chest away from

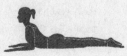

your mat. Press down on the tops of your feet and traction your forearms back to stretch out your abdominals for 5 full breaths (30 seconds).

5. **Plank Pose:** Inhale, Plank Pose—keep your knees on the ground at first, lift your hips, then lift your knees in line with your hips. Keep your core engaged for 5 full breaths. Create one line of energy from your heels to the top of your head (30 seconds).

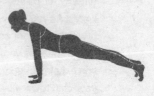

6. **Downward-Facing Dog:** Send your hips up high and fold your torso towards your thighs. Separate your hands shoulder width distance and your feet hip width distance and sink your heels towards your mat for 7 full breaths. Spread your fingers wide and press your chest towards your thighs (45 seconds).

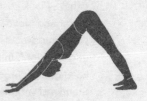

7. **Bridge Pose:** Lie all the way down on your back and place the soles of your feet on your mat. Inhale, Bridge Pose— peel your hips away from the mat and press your chest up and back. As you exhale, shimmy your shoulders underneath you and maybe gently join your hands for 5 breaths (30 seconds).

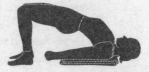

8. **Basic Relaxation Pose:** Slowly roll on your back one vertebra at a time, then extend your legs out long and arms long down by your sides, palms facing up. Gently close your eyes and relax for 5 minutes or more.

ENERGY SEQUENCE 4

1. **Mountain Pose:** Inhale—sweep your arms overhead, ground down through the four corners of your feet, engage your core, and make this an active pose for 5 full breaths (30 seconds).

2. **Standing Forward Bend:** Take one more breath in Mountain then exhale, Standing Forward Bend—bring your palms through heart center as you fold your torso towards your thighs and release your fingertips to your mat. Take 5 full breaths while allowing your head to hang heavy, then bend into one knee and then the next to warm up your hamstrings (30 seconds).

3. **Standing Half Forward Bend:** Inhale—place your palms on your shins or thighs, create a flat back, and breathe here for 5 full breaths. Work to parallel your torso to your mat and draw your shoulder blades together and down your back. Keep your gaze straight down (30 seconds).

4. **Plank Pose:** Exhale, Plank Pose—plant your palms shoulder width distance apart, step your feet straight back hip width distance apart, and keep your

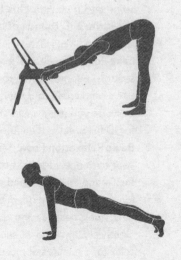

core engaged for 5 full breaths. Create one line of energy from your heels to the top of your head (30 seconds).

5. **Locust Pose:** Inhale in Plank Pose then exhale as you lower all the way down to your belly. Bring your arms out to a T and inhale in Locust Pose—peel your arms, chest, and thighs away from the mat and keep your legs engaged. Take 3 breaths here (20 seconds).

6. **Cat-Cow:** Place your shoulders directly under your palms, your hips over your knees. As you inhale, send your belly towards the floor and your tailbone up, and gaze towards the ceiling. As you exhale, round your spine and tuck your chin towards your chest. Take 10 rounds of breath here (1 minute).

7. **Easy Pose:** Come to take a comfortable seat on your mat. Come to your buttock bones and cross your shins. Bring your palms to your thighs and close your eyes for 10 full breaths (1 minute).

8. **Basic Relaxation Pose:** Slowly roll on your back one vertebra at a time for Basic Relaxation Pose—extend your legs out long and arms long down by your sides, palms facing up. Gently close your eyes and relax for 5 minutes or more.

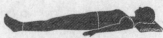

RELAXATION SEQUENCE 1

1. **Child's Pose:** Bring your big toes to touch and bring your knees to the edges of your mat. Crawl your fingertips towards the top of your mat and let your hips sink towards your heels. Let your forehead rest on your mat and spread your fingers wide. Breathe here for 10 full breaths (1 minute).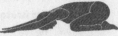

2. **Easy Pose:** Come to take a comfortable seat on your mat. Come to your buttock bones and cross your shins. Bring your palms to your thighs and close your eyes for 10 full breaths (1 minute).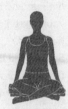

3. **Seated Straight-Leg Forward Bend:** Extend your legs out long in front of you, then inhale—find Mountain in your upper body, then exhale, Seated Straight-Leg Forward Bend—hinge at your hips and fold your torso towards your thighs. Bend your knees any amount and take 10 full breaths here (1 minute).

4. **Sideways Wide-Angle Pose:** Inhale, rise back up and reach your arms overhead, open your legs out wide, and exhale, Sideways Wide-Angle—pivot your torso towards your right leg and fold over your leg. Bend your leg any amount and breathe here for 5 full breaths (30 seconds).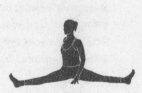

5. Repeat **Sideways Wide-Angle Pose** on the left side.

6. **Seated Wide-Angle Pose:** Keep your legs where they are, walk your hands out in front of you, and bend your knees any amount. Bow your head towards your mat and breathe here for 10 full breaths (1 minute).

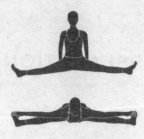

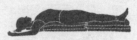

7. **Restorative Bridge Pose:** Come to lie all the way down on your back and place the soles of your feet on your mat. Inhale Restorative Bridge—peel your hips away from the mat and put a block underneath your sacrum for 10 full breaths (1 minute).

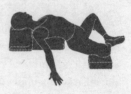

8. **Supported Bound Angle Pose:** Bring the soles of your feet to touch, and splay your knees out wide. Extend your arms out long by your sides, palms facing up, for 10 full breaths (1 minute).

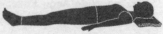

9. **Basic Relaxation Pose:** Gently bring your knees into your chest, then extend your legs out long and arms long down by your sides, palms facing up, for Basic Relaxation Pose— slowly close your eyes and relax for 5 minutes or more.

RELAXATION SEQUENCE 2

1. **Basic Relaxation Pose:** Lie on your
   back for Basic Relaxation Pose.
   Extend your legs out long and arms
   long down by your sides, palms
   facing up. Gently close your eyes and
   relax for 5 minutes or more.

   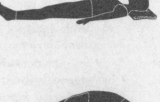

2. **Seated Straight-Leg Forward Bend:**
   Bring your knees into your chest and
   rock and roll all the way up to your
   buttock bones. Extend your legs out
   long in front of you, then inhale—
   find Mountain in your upper body then
   exhale, Seated Straight-Leg Forward Bend—
   hinge at your hips and fold your torso towards
   your thighs. Bend your knees any amount and
   take 10 full breaths here (1 minute).

   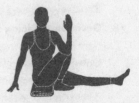

3. **Sage Twist:** Bend your right knee and
   place your heel as close as you can to
   your buttock bone. Inhale and then
   exhale, Sage Twist—rotate your torso
   to the right and wrap your left arm
   around your bent knee for 10 full breaths
   (1 minute).

   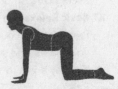

4. Repeat **Sage Twist** on the other side.

5. **Cat-Cow:** Place your shoulders directly
   under your palms, your hips over your
   knees. As you inhale, send your belly
   towards the floor and your tailbone up, and
   gaze towards the ceiling. As you exhale,

round your spine and tuck your chin towards your chest. Take 10 rounds of breath here (1 minute).

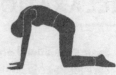

6. **Downward-Facing Dog:** Send your hips up high and fold your torso towards your thighs. Separate your hands shoulder width distance and your feet hip width distance and sink your heels towards your mat for 7 full breaths. Spread your fingers wide and press your chest towards your thighs (45 seconds).

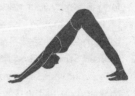

7. **Pigeon Pose:** Inhale, your right leg high; exhale, Pigeon Pose—bring your right knee to your right wrist, and work to parallel your shin to the top of your mat. Inhale, find length in your spine; exhale, walk your hands out in front of you, and fold over your front leg. Take 10 full breaths here (1 minute).

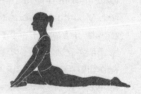

8. **Downward-Facing Dog:** Bring your right leg back to meet your left leg for Downward-Facing Dog—send your hips up and back and breathe here for 3 breaths (20 seconds).

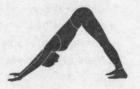

9. Repeat **Pigeon Pose** and **Downward-Facing Dog** on the left side.

10. **Basic Relaxation Pose:** Step your feet between your hands, bend your knees, and sink your hips all the way down to your mat for Basic Relaxation Pose. Gently close your eyes and relax for 5 minutes or more.

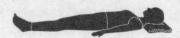

RELAXATION SEQUENCE 3

1. **Supported Bound Angle Pose:** Bring the soles of your feet to touch, and splay your knees out wide. Extend your arms out long by your sides, palms facing up, for 10 full breaths (1 minute).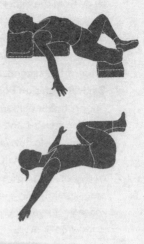

2. **Belly Twist:** Bring your knees into your chest, then stack your knees directly over your hips and bring your shins parallel to your mat. Inhale; then exhale, Belly Twist—bring your knees all the way on the floor so they are stacked on top of one another. Offer your right arm and maybe your gaze to the right and breathe here for 10 full breaths (1 minute).

3. Repeat **Supported Bound Angle Pose** and **Belly Twist** (in that order) on the other side.

4. **Restorative Bridge Pose:** Come to lie all the way down on your back and place the soles of your feet on your mat. Inhale Restorative Bridge—peel your hips away from the mat and put a block underneath your sacrum for 10 full breaths (1 minute).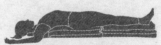

5. **Supported Legs Up the Wall:** Lower your back all the way to the floor, then draw your knees into your chest, then send your feet straight up towards the ceiling. Your feet should be stacked directly on top of your hips. Breathe here for 10 full breaths (1 minute).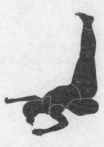

6. **Supported Shoulderstand:** Keep your legs where they are and lift your hips away from the mat. Place your palms on your lower back, scoot your elbows in towards one another, and find space between your chin and chest for 5 full breaths (30 seconds).

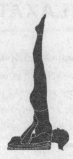

7. **Basic Relaxation Pose:** Come out of Supported Shoulderstand the same way you came into it and come to lie on your back for Basic Relaxation Pose. Extend your legs out long and arms long down by your sides, palms facing up. Gently close your eyes and relax for 5 minutes or more.

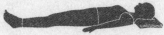

RELAXATION SEQUENCE 4

1. **Basic Relaxation Pose:** Lie on your back for Basic Relaxation Pose. Extend your legs out long and arms long down by your sides, palms facing up. Gently close your eyes and relax for 5 minutes or more.

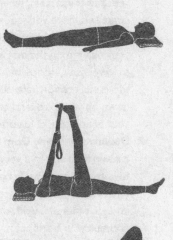

2. **Reclining Hand-to-Big-Toe Pose I:** Send your right foot straight up and use a strap around the arch of your foot to pull your leg towards your torso for a deep hamstring stretch for 5 full breaths (30 seconds).

3. **Reclining Hand-to-Big-Toe Pose II:** Grab hold of the strap with your right hand and begin to draw your foot to the right side of the room. Keep your pelvis on the floor and breathe here for 5 full breaths (30 seconds).

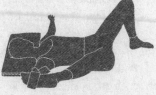

4. Repeat **Reclining Hand-to-Big-Toe Pose I** and **II** (in that order) on the left side.

5. **Bound Angle Pose:** Bring both knees into your chest and rock and roll all the way up to your buttock bones. Bring the soles of your feet to touch, and splay your knees out wide. Close your eyes and find a straight spine for 5 full breaths (30 seconds).

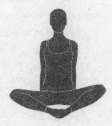

6. **Reclining Hero Pose:** Come to sit on your shins and bring your knees to touch. Bring your ankles apart and move your calves to the outside of your thighs. Softly lower your pelvis onto the mat and begin to lower your elbows behind you. If this is still comfortable, come to lie all the way down on your back and bring your arms above your head. Take 10 full breaths here (1 minute).

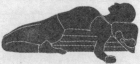

7. **Downward-Facing Dog:** Send your hips up high and fold your torso towards your thighs. Separate your hands shoulder width distance and your feet hip width distance and sink your heels towards your mat for 7 full breaths. Spread your fingers wide and press your chest towards your thighs (45 seconds).

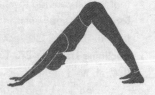

8. **Pigeon Pose:** Inhale, your right leg high; exhale, Pigeon Pose—bring your right knee to your right wrist, and work to parallel your shin to the top of your mat. Inhale, find length in your spine; exhale, walk your hands out in front of you, and fold over your front leg. Take 10 full breaths here (1 minute).

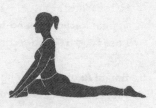

9. **Downward-Facing Dog:** Bring your right leg to meet your left leg for Downward-Facing Dog—send your hips up and back and breathe here for 5 breaths (30 seconds).

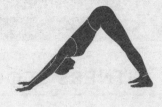

10. Repeat **Pigeon** and **Downward-Facing Dog** on the left side.

11. **Basic Relaxation Pose:** Step your feet between your hands, bend your knees, and sink your hips all the way down to your mat for Basic Relaxation Pose. Slowly roll on your back one vertebra at a time, then extend your legs out long and arms long down by your sides, palms facing up. Gently close your eyes and relax for 5 minutes or more.

FITNESS SEQUENCE 1

1. **Downward-Facing Dog:** Send your hips up high and fold your torso towards your thighs. Separate your hands shoulder width distance and your feet hip width and sink your heels towards your mat for 7 full breaths. Spread your fingers wide and press your chest towards your thighs (45 seconds).

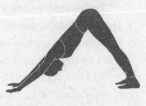

2. **Standing Forward Bend:** Inhale, look between your hands, then exhale, Standing Forward Bend—step your feet between your palms (big toes touching) and let your torso hang from your hips. Take 5 full breaths while allowing your head to hang heavy, then bend into one knee and then the next to warm up your hamstrings (30 seconds).

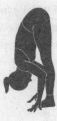

3. **Standing Half Forward Bend:** Inhale— place your palms on your shins or thighs, create a flat back, and breathe here for 5 full breaths. Work to parallel your torso to your mat and draw your shoulder blades together and down your back. Keep your gaze straight down (30 seconds).

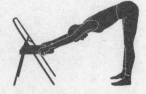

4. **Chair Pose/Fierce Warrior:** Inhale, bend your knees deeply, then rise up and reach your arms straight overhead. Be strong in your base and heavy in your heels, and squeeze your thighs together. Knit your low ribs in and relax your shoulders away from your ears for 5 full breaths (30 seconds).

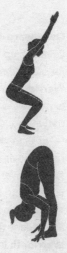

5. **Standing Forward Bend:** Inhale in Chair Pose then exhale, Standing Forward Bend—hinge at your hips and release your fingertips to your mat for 3 breaths (20 seconds).

6. **Standing Half Forward Bend:** Inhale—create a flat back and breathe here for 2 full breaths (10 seconds).

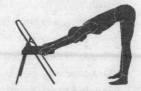

7. **Plank Pose:** Exhale, Plank Pose— plant your palms shoulder width distance apart, step your feet straight back hip width distance apart, and keep your core engaged for 5 full breaths. Create one line of energy from your heels to the top of your head (30 seconds).

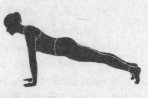

8. **Upward-Facing Dog:** Inhale— open your chest forward as you flip onto the tops of your feet. Breathe here for 2 breaths (10 seconds) and press down on the tops of your feet to engage your knees and thighs enough to lift them away from your mat.

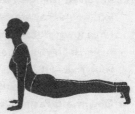

9. **Downward-Facing Dog:** Exhale, send your hips up and back, and breathe here for 5 breaths (30 seconds).

10. **Warrior I:** Inhale and raise your right leg high, then exhale and place your foot between your palms. Inhale, Warrior I—ground your back heel down, then rise up to stand and reach your arms straight overhead. Work to square your hips to the front the best you can and breathe here for 5 full breaths (30 seconds).

11. **Warrior II:** Inhale in Warrior I then exhale to Warrior II—adjust your feet, open up to the left side of the room, and bring your arms in line with your shoulders for 5 full breaths (30 seconds).

12. **Triangle Pose:** Inhale and straighten your front knee; exhale and reach your front arm forward and down, your left arm up to the ceiling. Work to stack your shoulders directly on top of one another and breathe here for 5 full breaths (30 seconds).

13. **Revolved Triangle Pose:** Keep your legs where they are and rotate your torso towards the right side of the room. Bring your left arm down towards your front foot and your right arm up to the ceiling for 5 breaths (30 seconds).

14. **Downward-Facing Dog:** Inhale in

Revolved Triangle then exhale, Downward-Facing Dog—plant your palms and step your feet back as you send your hips up and back. Breathe here for 5 breaths (30 seconds).

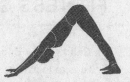

15. Repeat **Warrior I, Warrior II, Triangle Pose, Revolved Triangle Pose,** and **Downward-Facing Dog** (in that order) on the left side.

16. **Basic Relaxation Pose:** Step your feet between your hands, bend your knees and sink your hips all the way down to your mat for Basic Relaxation Pose. Slowly roll on your back one vertebra at a time, then extend your legs out long and arms long down by your sides, palms facing up. Gently close your eyes and relax for 5 minutes or more.

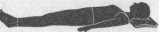

FITNESS SEQUENCE 2

1. **Child's Pose:** Bring your big toes to touch and bring your knees to the edges of your mat. Crawl your fingertips towards the top of your mat and let your hips sink towards your heels. Let your forehead rest on your mat and spread your fingers wide. Breathe here for 10 full breaths (1 minute).

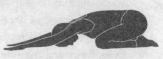

2. **Cat-Cow:** Place your shoulders directly under your palms, your hips over your knees. As you inhale, send your belly towards the floor and your tailbone up and gaze towards the ceiling. As you exhale, round your spine and tuck your chin towards your chest. Take 10 rounds of breath here (1 minute).

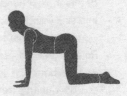

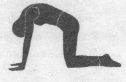

3. **Downward-Facing Dog:** Send your hips up high and fold your torso towards your thighs. Separate your hands shoulder width distance and your feet hip width distance and sink your heels towards your mat for 7 full breaths. Spread your fingers wide and press your chest towards your thighs (45 seconds).

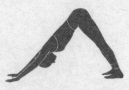

4. **Standing Forward Bend:** Inhale, look between your hands, then exhale, Standing Forward Bend—step your feet between your palms (big toes touching) and let your torso hang from your hips. Take 5 full breaths while allowing your head to hang heavy, then bend into one knee and then the next to warm up your hamstrings (30 seconds).

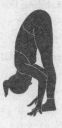

5. **Standing Half Forward Bend:** Inhale—place your palms on your shins or thighs, create a flat back, and breathe here for 5 full breaths. Work to parallel your torso to your mat and draw your shoulder blades together and down your back. Keep your gaze straight down (30 seconds).

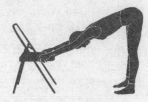

6. **Standing Forward Bend:** Inhale in Standing Half Forward Bend, then exhale, Standing Forward Bend—release your torso and fingertips to your mat for 5 breaths (30 seconds).

7. **Chair Pose/Fierce Warrior:** Inhale, bend your knees deeply, then rise up and reach your arms straight overhead. Be strong in your base and heavy in your heels, and squeeze your thighs together. Knit your low ribs in and relax your shoulders away from your ears for 5 full breaths (30 seconds).

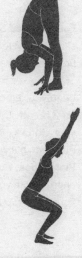

8. **Standing Forward Bend:** Exhale, release your torso and fingertips to your mat for 3 breaths (20 seconds).

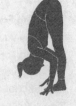

9. **Standing Half Forward Bend:** Inhale— place your palms on your shins or thighs, create a flat back, and breathe here for 2 full breaths. Work to parallel your torso to your mat and draw your shoulder blades together and down your back. Keep your gaze straight down (10 seconds).

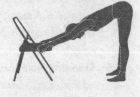

10. **Plank Pose:** Exhale, Plank Pose—plant your palms shoulder width distance apart, step your feet straight back hip width distance apart, and keep your core engaged for 5 full breaths. Create one line of energy from your heels to the top of your head (30 seconds).

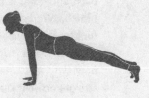

11. **Four-Limbed Staff Pose:** Inhale and shift your weight forward in Plank Pose then exhale, Four-Limbed Staff—lower halfway down and bend your elbows up to 90 degrees for 2 breaths (10 seconds). Keep your elbows pinned into your low ribs and your gaze down.

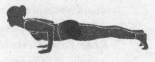

12. **Plank Pose:** Create one line of energy from your heels to the top of your head (30 seconds).

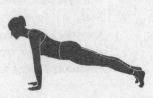

13. **Four-Limbed Staff Pose:** Inhale and shift your weight forward in Plank Pose then exhale, Four-Limbed Staff again—lower halfway down and bend your elbows up to 90 degrees for 2 breaths (10 seconds). Keep your elbows pinned into your low ribs and your gaze down.

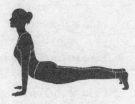

14. **Upward-Facing Dog:** Inhale—open your chest forward as you flip onto the tops of your feet. Breathe here for 3 breaths (20 seconds) and press down on the tops of your feet to engage your knees and thighs enough to lift them away from your mat.

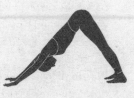

15. **Downward-Facing Dog:** Exhale, send your hips up and back, and breathe here for 5 breaths (30 seconds).

16. **Basic Relaxation Pose:** Step your feet between your hands, bend your knees, and sink your hips all the way down to your mat for Basic Relaxation Pose. Slowly roll on your back one vertebra at a time, then extend your legs out long and arms long down by your sides, palms facing up. Gently close your eyes and relax for 5 minutes or more.

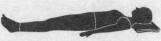

FITNESS SEQUENCE 3

1. **Downward-Facing Dog:** Send your hips up high and fold your torso towards your thighs. Separate your hands shoulder width distance and your feet hip width distance and sink your heels towards your mat for 7 full breaths. Spread your fingers wide and press your chest towards your thighs (45 seconds).

2. **Equestrian/Lunge Pose:** Inhale and raise your right leg high; exhale, Equestrian/Lunge—place your foot between your palms and bring your back knee down to your mat. Send your chest and hips forward, and gaze straight ahead for 5 breaths (30 seconds).

3. **Warrior I:** Inhale, ground your back heel down, then rise up to stand and reach your arms straight overhead. Work to square your hips to the front the best you can and breathe here for 5 full breaths (30 seconds).

4. **Warrior II:** Inhale Warrior II—ground your back heel down, rise up, and extend your arms to the front and back of the room. Open your left hip and bend into your front knee up to 90 degrees for 5 full breaths (30 seconds).

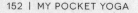

5. **Triangle Pose:** Inhale and straighten your front knee; exhale and reach your front arm forward and down, your left arm up to the ceiling. Work to stack your shoulders directly on top of one another and breathe here for 5 full breaths (30 seconds).

6. **Intense Side Stretch Pose:** Inhale and rise back up to stand and reach your arms up; keep your legs where they are and pivot your torso towards your front foot. Shorten your stance with all 10 toes pointing forward. Exhale, Intense Side Stretch—hinge at your hips and fold your torso towards your front leg. Soften your front knee and place your hands on either side of your front foot. Breathe here for 5 breaths (30 seconds).

7. **Extended Side Angle Pose:** Inhale in Warrior II then exhale, Extended Side Angle—reach your front arm forward and then down, and reach your back arm up to the ceiling. Continue to reach up towards your top fingertips for 5 breaths (30 seconds).

8. **Warrior II:** Inhale, keep your legs as they are, and rise up for 5 full breaths (30 seconds).

9. **Plank Pose:** Exhale, Plank Pose—plant your palms shoulder width distance apart, step your feet straight back hip width distance apart, and keep your core engaged for 5 full breaths. Create one line of energy from your heels to the top of your head (30 seconds).

10. **Four-Limbed Staff Pose:** Inhale and shift your weight forward in Plank Pose then exhale, Four-Limbed Staff—lower halfway down and bend your elbows up to 90 degrees for 2 breaths (10 seconds). Keep your elbows pinned into your low ribs and your gaze down.

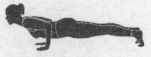

11. **Upward-Facing Dog:** Inhale—open your chest forward as you flip onto the tops of your feet. Breathe here for 5 breaths (30 seconds) and press down on the tops of your feet to engage your knees and thighs enough to lift them away from your mat.

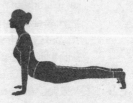

12. **Downward-Facing Dog:** Exhale, send your hips up and back, and breathe here for 5 breaths (30 seconds).

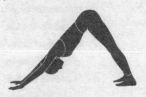

13. Repeat **Equestrian/Lunge Pose, Warrior I, Warrior II, Triangle Pose, Intense Side Stretch Pose, Extended Side Angle Pose, Warrior II, Plank Pose, Four-Limbed Staff Pose, Upward-Facing Dog,** and **Downward-Facing Dog** (in that order) on the left side.

14. **Basic Relaxation Pose:** Step your feet between your hands, bend your knees, and sink your hips all the way down to your mat for Basic Relaxation Pose. Slowly roll on your back one vertebra at a time, then extend your legs out long and arms long down by your sides, palms facing up. Gently close your eyes and relax for 5 minutes or more.

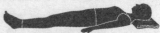

FITNESS SEQUENCE 4

1. **Mountain Pose:** Inhale—sweep your arms overhead, ground down through the four corners of your feet, engage your core, and make this an active pose for 5 full breaths (30 seconds).

2. **Standing Backbend Pose:** Inhale in Mountain then exhale, Standing Backbend—bend at your elbows, open your chest to the ceiling, and engage your abdominals for 3 full breaths (20 seconds).

3. **Mountain Pose:** Inhale, rise back up to Mountain for 2 breaths. Squeeze your thighs together, tuck your tailbone down, and relax your shoulders away from your ears (15 seconds).

4. **Standing Forward Bend:** Take one more breath in Mountain then exhale, Standing Forward Bend—bring your palms through heart center as you fold your torso towards your thighs and release your fingertips to your mat. Take 5 full breaths allowing your head to hang heavy, and bend into one knee and then the next to warm up your hamstrings (30 seconds).

5. **Standing Half Forward Bend:** Inhale—place your palms on your shins or thighs, create a flat back, and breathe here for 5 full breaths. Work to parallel your torso to your mat and draw your shoulder blades together and down your back. Keep your gaze straight down (30 seconds).

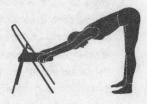

6. **Plank Pose:** Exhale, Plank Pose—plant your palms shoulder width distance apart, step your feet straight back hip width distance apart, and keep your core engaged for 5 full breaths. Create one line of energy from your heels to the top of your head (30 seconds).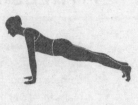

7. **Salute with Eight Parts or Points:** Inhale in Plank Pose then exhale to Salute with Eight Parts or Points—bring your knees to your mat, then send your hips up high and bend at your elbows to bring your chin to your mat. Breathe here for 3 full breaths (20 seconds).

8. **Plank Pose:** Inhale to Plank Pose—create one line of energy from your heels to the top of your head for 3 full breaths (20 seconds).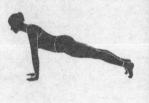

9. **Four-Limbed Staff Pose:** Inhale and shift your weight forward in Plank Pose then exhale, Four-Limbed Staff—lower halfway down and bend your elbows up to 90 degrees for 2 breaths (10 seconds). Keep your elbows pinned into your low ribs and your gaze down.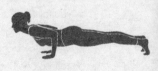

10. **Upward-Facing Dog:** Inhale—open your chest forward as you flip onto the tops of your feet. Breathe here for 3 breaths (20 seconds) and press down on the tops of your feet to engage your knees and thighs enough to lift them away from your mat.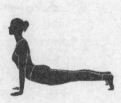

11. **Downward-Facing Dog:** Send your hips up high and fold your torso towards your thighs. Separate your hands shoulder width distance and your feet hip width distance, and sink your heels towards your mat for 7 full breaths. Spread your fingers wide and press your chest towards your thighs (45 seconds).

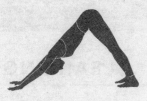

12. **Basic Relaxation Pose:** Step your feet between your hands, bend your knees, and sink your hips all the way down to your mat for Basic Relaxation Pose. Slowly roll on your back one vertebra at a time, then extend your legs out long and arms long down by your sides, palms facing up. Gently close your eyes and relax for 5 minutes or more.

CLEANSING SEQUENCE 1

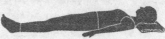

1. **Basic Relaxation Pose:** Lie on your back for Basic Relaxation Pose. Extend your legs out long and arms long down by your sides, palms facing up. Gently close your eyes and relax for 5 minutes or more.

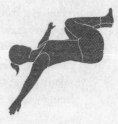

2. **Belly Twist:** Bring your knees into your chest, then stack your knees directly over your hips and bring your shins parallel to your mat. Inhale; then exhale, Belly Twist—bring your knees all the way on the floor so they are stacked on top of one another. Offer your right arm and maybe your gaze to the right and breathe here for 10 full breaths (1 minute).

3. Repeat **Belly Twist** on the left side.

4. **Downward-Facing Dog:** Roll up to a seat and place your palms on your mat, send your hips up high, and fold your torso towards your thighs for Downward-Facing Dog—separate your hands shoulder width distance and your feet hip width distance, and sink your heels towards your mat for 7 full breaths. Spread your fingers wide and press your chest towards your thighs (45 seconds).

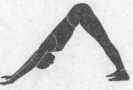

5. **Extended Side Angle Pose:** Inhale and raise your right leg high, then exhale as you step your foot between your hands. Inhale Extended Side Angle—keep your right hand down and reach your left arm up towards the ceiling, stacking your shoulders on top of one another for 5 full breaths (30 seconds).

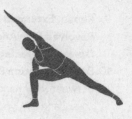

6. **Revolved Side Angle Pose:** Inhale in Extended Side Angle then exhale, Revolved Side Angle—keep your legs where they are and twist your torso towards the right side of the room. Send your right arm straight up and your left arm down. Engage your core and breathe here for 5 full breaths (30 seconds).

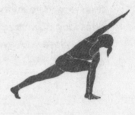

7. **Plank Pose:** Inhale in Revolved Side Angle then exhale, Plank Pose—plant your palms shoulder width distance apart, step your feet straight back hip width distance apart, and keep your core engaged for 5 full breaths. Create one line of energy from your heels to the top of your head (30 seconds).

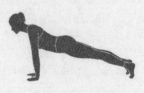

8. **Downward-Facing Dog:** Exhale, send your hips up and back, and breathe here for 5 breaths (30 seconds).

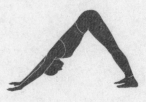

9. Repeat **Extended Side Angle Pose** and **Revolved Side Angle Pose, Plank Pose,** and **Downward-Facing Dog** on other side.

10. **Basic Relaxation Pose:** Step your feet between your hands, bend your knees, and sink your hips all the way down to your mat for Basic Relaxation Pose. Slowly roll on your back one vertebra at a time, then extend your legs out long and arms long down by your sides, palms facing up. Gently close your eyes and relax for 5 minutes or more.

CLEANSING SEQUENCE 2

1. **Easy Pose:** Take a comfortable seat on your mat. Come to your buttock bones and cross your shins. Bring your palms to your thighs and close your eyes for 10 full breaths (1 minute).

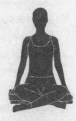

2. **Seated Straight-Leg Forward Bend:** Extend your legs out long in front of you, then inhale—find Mountain in your upper body then exhale, Seated Straight-Leg Forward Bend—hinge at your hips and fold your torso towards your thighs. Bend your knees any amount and take 10 full breaths here (1 minute).

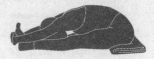

3. **Sideways Wide-Angle Pose:** Inhale, rise back up and reach your arms overhead, open your legs out wide, and exhale, Sideways Wide-Angle—pivot your torso towards your right leg and fold over your leg. Bend your leg any amount and breathe here for 5 full breaths (30 seconds).

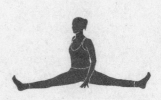

4. Repeat **Sideways Wide-Angle Pose** on the left side.

5. **Sage Twist:** Bend your right knee and place your heel as close as you can to your buttock bone. Inhale and then exhale, Sage Twist—rotate your torso to the right and wrap your left arm around your bent knee for 10 full breaths (1 minute).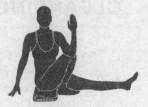

6. Repeat **Sage Twist** on the left side.

7. **Basic Relaxation Pose:** Come to lie on your back for Basic Relaxation Pose. Extend your legs out long and arms long down by your sides, palms facing up. Gently close your eyes and relax for 5 minutes or more.

CLEANSING SEQUENCE 3

1. **Downward-Facing Dog:** Send your hips up high and fold your torso towards your thighs. Separate your hands shoulder width distance and your feet hip width distance, and sink your heels towards your mat for 7 full breaths. Spread your fingers wide and press your chest towards your thighs (45 seconds).

2. **Warrior II:** Inhale and raise your right leg high, then exhale and place your foot between your hands. Inhale Warrior II—ground your back heel down, rise up, and extend your arms to the front and back of the room. Open your left hip and bend into your front knee up to 90 degrees for 5 full breaths (30 seconds).

3. **Triangle Pose:** Inhale and straighten your front knee; exhale and reach your front arm forward and down, your left arm up to the ceiling. Work to stack your shoulders directly on top of one another and breathe here for 5 full breaths (30 seconds).

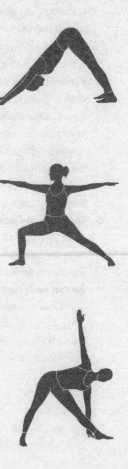

4. **Revolved Triangle Pose:** Keep your legs where they are and rotate your torso towards the right side of the room. Bring your left arm down towards your front foot and your right arm up to the ceiling for 5 breaths (30 seconds).

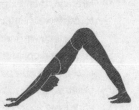

5. **Plank Pose:** Inhale in Revolved Triangle then exhale, Plank Pose—plant your palms shoulder width distance apart, step your feet straight back hip width distance apart, and keep your core engaged for 5 full breaths. Create one line of energy from your heels to the top of your head (30 seconds).

6. **Downward-Facing Dog:** Exhale, send your hips up and back, and breathe here for 5 breaths (30 seconds).

7. Repeat **Warrior II, Triangle Pose, Revolved Triangle Pose, Plank Pose,** and **Downward-Facing Dog** (in that order) on the left side.

8. **Basic Relaxation Pose:** Step your feet between your hands, bend your knees, and sink your hips all the way down to your mat for Basic Relaxation Pose. Slowly roll on your back one vertebra at a time, then extend your legs out long and arms long down by your sides, palms facing up. Gently close your eyes and relax for 5 minutes or more.

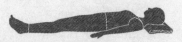

CLEANSING SEQUENCE 4

1. **Child's Pose:** Bring your big toes to touch and bring your knees to the edges of your mat. Crawl your fingertips towards the top of your mat and let your hips sink towards your heels. Let your forehead rest on your mat and spread your fingers wide. Breathe here for 10 full breaths (1 minute).

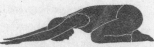

2. **Downward-Facing Dog:** Send your hips up high and fold your torso towards your thighs. Separate your hands shoulder width distance and your feet hip width distance, and sink your heels towards your mat for 7 full breaths. Spread your fingers wide and press your chest towards your thighs (45 seconds).

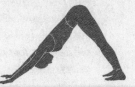

3. **Warrior I:** Inhale and raise your right leg high, then exhale and place your foot between your palms. Inhale Warrior I—ground your back heel down, then rise up to stand and reach your arms straight overhead. Work to square your hips to the front the best you can and breathe here for 5 full breaths (30 seconds).

4. **Intense Side Stretch Pose:** Shorten your stance and point all 10 toes straight forward. Inhale to find length in your spine, then exhale, Intense Side Stretch—hinge at your hips and fold your torso towards

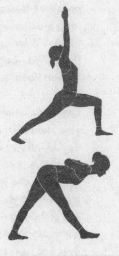

your front leg. Soften your front knee and place your hands on either side of your front foot. Breathe here for 5 breaths (30 seconds).

5. **Wide-Legged Forward Bend:** Move your torso so it is centered between your legs. Place your fingertips on the floor (or your palms, if flexible), shoulder width apart, either in line with the toes or in front of the toes. Breathe here for 5 breaths (30 seconds).

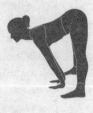

6. **Pigeon Pose:** Inhale and raise your right leg high; exhale, Pigeon Pose—bring your right knee to your right wrist, and work to parallel your shin to the top of your mat. Inhale, find length in your spine; exhale, walk your hands out in front of you and fold over your front leg. Take 10 full breaths here (1 minute).

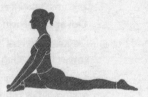

7. **Downward-Facing Dog:** Exhale, send your hips up and back, and breathe here for 5 breaths (30 seconds).

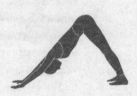

8. Repeat **Warrior I, Intense Side Stretch Pose, Wide-Legged Forward Bend, Pigeon Pose,** and **Downward-Facing Dog** (in that order) on the left side.

9. **Basic Relaxation Pose:** Step your feet between your hands, bend your knees, and sink your hips all the way down to your mat for Basic Relaxation Pose. Slowly roll on your back one vertebra at a time, then extend your legs out long and arms long down by your sides, palms facing up. Gently close your eyes and relax for 5 minutes or more.

FOCUS SEQUENCE 1

1. **Mountain Pose:** Inhale—sweep your arms overhead, ground down through the four corners of your feet, engage your core, and make this an active pose for 5 full breaths (30 seconds).
2. **Standing Backbend Pose:** Inhale in Mountain then exhale, Standing Backbend—bend at your elbows, open your chest to the ceiling, and engage your abdominals for 3 full breaths (20 seconds).
3. **Mountain Pose:** Inhale, rise back up to Mountain for 2 breaths. Squeeze your thighs together, tuck your tailbone down, and relax your shoulders away from your ears (10 seconds).
4. **Eagle Pose:** Wrap your right arm under your left and bring your palms to touch. Shift your weight into your left leg, then wrap your right leg over your left leg and work to wrap your foot around your calf. Squeeze everything into the midline of your body and find a non-moving point of focus to gaze at to improve your balance. Breathe here for 5 full breaths (30 seconds).

5. **Mountain Pose:** Inhale, unwind your arms and legs, and rise back up to Mountain for 2 breaths (10 seconds).

6. Repeat **Eagle Pose** and **Mountain Pose** on the left side.

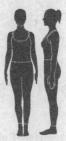

7. **Standing Forward Bend:** Take one more breath in Mountain then exhale, Standing Forward Bend—bring your palms through heart center as you fold your torso towards your thighs and release your fingertips to your mat. Take 5 full breaths while allowing your head to hang heavy, and bend into one knee and then the next to warm up your hamstrings (30 seconds).

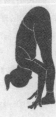

8. **Basic Relaxation Pose:** Step your feet between your hands, bend your knees, and sink your hips all the way down to your mat for Basic Relaxation Pose. Slowly roll on your back one vertebra at a time, then extend your legs out long and arms long down by your sides, palms facing up. Gently close your eyes and relax for 5 minutes or more.

FOCUS SEQUENCE 2

1. **Downward-Facing Dog:** Send your hips up high and fold your torso towards your thighs. Separate your hands shoulder width distance and your feet hip width distance, and sink your heels towards your mat for 7 full breaths. Spread your fingers wide and press your chest towards your thighs (45 seconds).

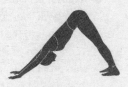

2. **Warrior II:** Inhale and raise your right leg high, then exhale and place your foot between your hands. Inhale, Warrior II—ground your back heel down, then rise up and extend your arms to the front and back of the room. Open your left hip and bend into your front knee up to 90 degrees for 5 full breaths (30 seconds).

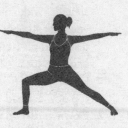

3. **Extended Side Angle Pose:** Inhale in Warrior II then exhale, Extended Side Angle—reach your front arm forward and then down, and reach your back arm up to the ceiling. Continue to reach up towards your top fingertips for 5 breaths (30 seconds).

4. **Half-Moon Pose:** Inhale in Extended Side Angle then exhale into Half-Moon—launch off your back foot and bring your back foot in line with your hips. Send your left arm up to the ceiling and your right arm down to the ground. Optionally,

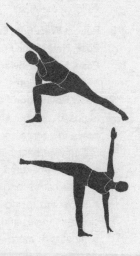

use a block under your right hand. Stack your shoulders on top of one another and find balance for 5 breaths (30 seconds).

5. **Warrior II:** Inhale, Warrior II—ground your back heel down, rise up, and extend your arms to the front and back of the room. Open your left hip and bend into your front knee up to 90 degrees for 5 full breaths (30 seconds).

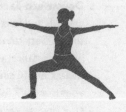

6. **Plank Pose:** Inhale in Warrior II then exhale, Plank Pose—plant your palms shoulder width distance apart, step your feet straight back hip width distance apart, and keep your core engaged for 5 full breaths. Create one line of energy from your heels to the top of your head (30 seconds).

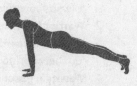

7. **Downward-Facing Dog:** Exhale, send your hips up and back, and breathe here for 5 breaths (30 seconds).

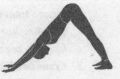

8. Repeat **Warrior II, Extended Side Angle Pose, Half-Moon Pose, Warrior II, Plank Pose,** and **Downward-Facing Dog** (in that order) on the left side.

9. **Basic Relaxation Pose:** Step your feet between your hands, bend your knees, and sink your hips all the way down to your mat for Basic Relaxation Pose. Slowly roll on your back one vertebra at a time, then extend your legs out long and arms long down by your sides, palms facing up. Gently close your eyes and relax for 5 minutes or more.

FOCUS SEQUENCE 3

1. **Mountain Pose:** Inhale—sweep your arms overhead, ground down through the four corners of your feet, engage your core, and make this an active pose for 5 full breaths. Squeeze your thighs together, tuck your tailbone down, and relax your shoulders away from your ears (30 seconds).

2. **Tree Pose:** Bring your right foot to the inside of your left leg, either on your calf or upper thigh, and open your right hip to send your knee to the right side of the room. Breathe here for 5 breaths (30 seconds).

3. **Mountain Pose:** Inhale, sweep your arms up, and release your foot to the mat for 2 breaths (15 seconds).

4. Repeat **Tree Pose** and **Mountain Pose** on the left side.

5. **Standing Forward Bend:** Bring your palms through heart center as you fold your torso towards your thighs and release your fingertips to your mat. Take 5 full breaths while allowing your head to hang heavy, and bend into one knee and then the next to warm up your hamstrings (30 seconds).

6. **Basic Relaxation Pose:** Step your feet between your hands, bend your knees, and sink your hips all the way down to your mat for Basic Relaxation Pose. Slowly roll on your back one vertebra at a time, then extend your legs out long and arms long down by your sides, palms facing up. Gently close your eyes and relax for 5 minutes or more.

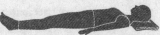

FOCUS SEQUENCE 4

1. **Child's Pose:** Bring your big toes to touch and bring your knees to the edges of your mat. Crawl your fingertips towards the top of your mat and let your hips sink towards your heels. Let your forehead rest on your mat and spread your fingers wide. Breathe here for 10 full breaths (1 minute).

2. **Downward-Facing Dog:** Send your hips up high and fold your torso towards your thighs. Separate your hands shoulder width distance and your feet hip width distance, and sink your heels towards your mat for 7 full breaths. Spread your fingers wide and press your chest towards your thighs (45 seconds).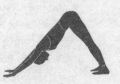

3. **Standing Forward Bend:** Inhale, look between your hands then exhale, Standing Forward Bend—step your feet between your palms (big toes touching), and let your torso hang from your hips. Take 5 full breaths while allowing your head to hang heavy, and bend into one knee and then the next to warm up your hamstrings (30 seconds).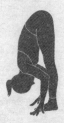

4. **Standing Half Forward Bend:** Inhale— place your palms on your shins or thighs, create a flat back, and breathe for 5 full breaths. Work to parallel your torso to your mat and draw your shoulder blades together and down your back. Keep your gaze straight down (30 seconds).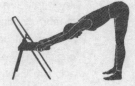

5. **Mountain Pose:** Inhale, rise back up to Mountain for 2 breaths. Squeeze your thighs together, tuck your tailbone down, and relax your shoulders away from your ears (10 seconds).

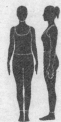

6. **Extended Hand on the Foot Pose:** Bring your left hand to your hip, then bring your left knee to your belly and grab for the outer edge of your right foot with your right hand. Extend your leg out in front of you and bend your knee any amount. If you're steady, then begin to open your leg out to the side and breathe for 5 full breaths (30 seconds).

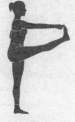

7. **Mountain Pose:** Inhale, sweep your arms up, and release your foot to the mat for 2 breaths (15 seconds).

8. Repeat **Extended Hand on the Foot Pose** and **Mountain Pose** on the left side.

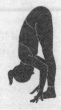

9. **Standing Forward Bend:** Take one more breath in Mountain then exhale, Standing Forward Bend—bring your palms through heart center as you fold your torso towards your thighs and release your fingertips to your mat. Take 5 full breaths while allowing your head to hang heavy, and bend into one knee and then the next to warm up your hamstrings (30 seconds).

10. **Basic Relaxation Pose:** Step your feet between your hands, bend your knees, and sink your hips all the way down to your mat for Basic Relaxation Pose. Slowly roll on your back one vertebra at a time, then extend your legs out long and arms long down by your sides, palms facing up. Gently close your eyes and relax for 5 minutes or more.

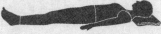

INDEX